MANAGING QUALITY
A Guide to
Monitoring and
Evaluating Nursing Services

MANAGING QUALITY

A Guide to
Monitoring and
Evaluating Nursing Services

JACQUELINE KATZ, RN, MS

Vice President, Professional Services
Resource Applications, Inc.

ELEANOR GREEN, RN, BSN

Senior Consultant
Quality Management Consulting Group
Resource Applications, Inc.

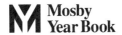

**Mosby
Year Book**

St. Louis Baltimore Boston Chicago London Philadelphia Sydney Toronto

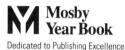

Mosby
Year Book
Dedicated to Publishing Excellence

Editor: N. Darlene Como
Editorial Assistant: Barbara Carroll
Project Supervisor: Lilliane Anstee
Book and Cover Design: Gail Morey Hudson

Printed in the United States of America

Mosby–Year Book, Inc.
11830 Westline Industrial Drive, St. Louis, MO 63146

Library of Congress Cataloging-in-Publication Data

Katz, Jacqueline.
    Managing quality : a guide to monitoring and evaluating nursing services / Jacqueline Katz, Eleanor Green.
       p.   cm.
    Includes bibliographical references and index.
    ISBN 0-8016-2620-X
    1. Nursing services—Evaluation. I. Green, Eleanor. II. Title.
    [DNLM: 1. Nursing Services—organization & administration—United States. 2. Quality Assurance, Health Care—United States—nurses' instruction. WY 100 K195m]
    RT85.5.K38 1992
    362.1′73′0287—dc20
    DNLM/DLC
    for Library of Congress
                                         91-25391
                                             CIP

93 94 95 96 VT/MY 9 8 7 6 5 4 3

To
Jay and Bunky
Two husbands who set the standard
against which all other husbands are measured.

ACKNOWLEDGMENTS

Many people have played many different and important roles in the development and publication of this book. Our special thanks go to:

Darlene Como, the world's most patient and forgiving editor, for her insight, understanding, and risk-taking.

Barbara Carroll for service above and beyond the call of duty and her constant enthusiasm.

Marley Bunce and Bette Householder for their flying fingers.

Our reviewers, Amy Kennedy, Peggy Reilly, and Toni Smith for their thought-provoking comments and suggestions and for keeping us on track.

Lilliane Anstee for keeping the project moving on schedule.

Bernice Heller for making our ideas and words come alive.

The many hospitals who believed in us and piloted our ideas and projects during the development phase.

The participants in our workshops for helping us to shape our ideas.

Our children: Sheri for keeping house; Scott for lending encouragement; a new daughter-in-law, Carol, for providing laughter; Lauren for learning her times tables by herself; Meryl for giving lots of hugs; and Evan for just being.

Our parents, Melvin and Ann Kedzior and Bill and Evelyn Postlewait, for being our best press agents.

Patricia Schroeder for her rare ability to encourage colleagues to reach new heights.

Our friend, Susan Sibiski, for tolerating (barely) our discussions about the "Q" and "N" words.

FOREWORD

Writing a book is an awesome task. It demands exceptional knowledge of the subject, an exemplary ability to communicate through the written word, time, and an unwavering commitment to complete the project through all of its inevitable ups and downs. Even in the best of situations, these requirements are daunting. Writing a book about managing quality in health care in the 1990s, however, defies the best of situations.

Changing regulations, shifting expectations, evolving approaches and terminology, and the generation of new knowledge typify the pursuit of quality today. To write a book about a rapidly changing field such as quality management in health care requires not only an understanding of the concepts but also participation in applying the ideas in clinical settings—to create the new vision and reality for quality programs.

This is an excellent book, written by noteworthy experts who have taught thousands of nurses and have assisted in implementing quality programs in numerous clinical agencies. *Managing Quality: A Guide to Monitoring and Evaluating Nursing Services* is one of the best books I have read on improving health care quality. It contains cutting-edge material and is based on the latest literature and extensive experience. It is relevant to health care in the 1990s in many clinical settings. Perhaps most compelling is the richness of practical examples given that are sure to clarify the material for readers and be of interest to them. One is virtually assured of gaining new insights and strategies from reading this book.

It has been said that knowledge is knowing a fact, but wisdom is knowing what to do with it. This book was written by two very wise women. Jackie Katz and Ellie Green have a keen understanding of quality management as it relates to the delivery of nursing care in today's health care organizations. In this book, the authors not only describe the concepts but also discuss how to use them effectively to improve practice, care, and organizational systems. They have articulated a vision for—as well as developed approaches to—the improvement of nursing care quality. This book reflects their knowledge, wisdom, and creativity.

As you read this book, its value and significance will become apparent. Irrespective of future changes in terminology, buzz words, and trends, the ideas and approaches presented in this book will stand the test of time. It is only through such contributions that we can hope to meet the complex and ever-changing needs for quality health care of the American public.

Patricia Schroeder, RN, MSN
Nursing Quality Consultant
Quality Care Concepts, Inc.

PREFACE

It is virtually impossible to be part of today's health care system and not appreciate the quality revolution that is taking place. Journal articles and books on quality abound. Billboard, radio, and magazine ads extol the quality of care delivered by various hospitals, HMOs, long-term care facilities, and home health agencies. From the board room to the medication room, discussions focus on quality issues.

The Tax Equity and Fiscal Responsibility Act (TEFRA) of 1982 and the subsequent prospective payment legislation had tremendous repercussions throughout the U.S. health care system. With so much attention being given to costs, one significant effect has been the need to revamp traditional quality approaches that focused previously on how services were delivered. The new emphasis in determining quality is on results produced by the services delivered. Services delivered are now being analyzed in relation to their ultimate effect on outcomes. "We've always done it that way" is no longer acceptable justification for specific interventions. In today's environment the critical response is that a particular action is essential to achieving the desired results.

The thrust of quality assurance in health care is changing dramatically. With the advent of the Joint Commission of Accreditation of Health Care Organizations' (Joint Commission's) Agenda for Change, the emphasis in quality monitoring has shifted from process to outcome. The monitoring and evaluation process must not only insure that an institution is able to deliver quality care but that the institution *does* deliver quality patient care. Moreover, economic survival dictates that the care also be delivered cost-effectively. This results orientation requires nursing to rethink its approach to monitoring its services.

Monitoring and evaluation activities in nursing must now be directed toward those priorities which have the greatest impact on results: the high-risk, high-volume, problem-prone, and high-cost aspects of nursing service that influence the balance between quality of care and cost containment.

The trend in nursing to decentralize quality assessment requires that each staff nurse become involved in monitoring and evaluating activities. Each nurse manager must have a mechanism for identifying and monitoring service priorities. The division of nursing must insure that the priorities are comprehensive in scope, addressing the high-risk, high-volume, problem-prone, and high-cost aspects of its service.

To assist the health care organization in monitoring the quality of its service, the Joint Commission designed a ten-step monitoring and evaluation process. This book provides a practical step-by-step plan for using the Joint Commission's ten-step process to create a quality assessment program. The book's new approach to the ten-step process is unique because it defines the clinical, professional, and administrative aspects of nursing as a service. The concept of nursing as a service business is revolutionary. Traditionally nursing has been defined by the clinical services it provides to patients. Yet, nursing serves many constituents: administration, patients, physicians, and staff. It must ensure customer satisfaction, quality results, and cost-effectiveness for each of its constituent groups. This book will assist the top, middle, or front-line manager or staff nurse to focus on the critical aspects of nursing as a business. It offers tools and techniques which will enable nurses to identify the clinical, professional, and administrative services which have the greatest impact on outcomes. The book also serves as a starting point for the transition to a statistically based quality management program. Statistical methods and statistical process control tools are explained to facilitate that transition.

The term *nurse manager* is used in this book to represent all nurses with administrative responsibilities for quality assessment and improvement. Included are directors and coordinators, staff nurses, department representatives, and clinical nurse specialists. Where quality is concerned, everyone is a manager.

Many nurse managers are responsible for managing services whose budget and staff are equal in size to those of other departments within the organization. For example, in a community hospital it is not uncommon for the coronary care unit to have a budget and staff equal to or greater than those of the physical therapy department. We, therefore, believe that rather than managing units, nurse managers manage service departments within the division of nursing. Therefore, throughout the text the term *nursing unit* has been replaced by *nursing department* and the term *division of nursing* is used to designate the entire nursing organization.

The Joint Commission's ten-step monitoring and evaluation process is purposely vague to allow for differing approaches. However, as a result, much confusion exists within nursing regarding how best to monitor and evaluate its service. What and how many things should I monitor? How often should I monitor each thing? How do I choose what to monitor? How do I set a threshold? These are just some of the questions frequently asked in health care institutions. This book is designed to take much of the guesswork out of the monitoring and evaluation process. It is a basic primer providing a concrete approach to implementing a quality management program integrating the Joint Commission's model and a framework for quality management called THE BLUEPRINT for Quality Management.

This new approach to monitoring and evaluation is a critical component of implementing a quality management initiative. It is a comprehensive system that can be used at the divisional, department, and bedside levels. It concentrates on problem identification and prevention and work efficiency in the high-risk, high-volume, problem-prone, and high-cost areas of nursing. It enables you to understand, monitor, and evaluate those aspects of service that are most critical to quality outcomes and that consume the most resources.

Using the practical tips, techniques, and tools included throughout the book and incorporating your department's characteristics and peculiarities, you can develop a comprehensive, statistically based monitoring and evaluation program congruent with the Joint Commission's ten-step process and the Agenda for Change.

The strategies and tools described in the book have been piloted, refined, and used successfully in hospitals throughout the United States and Canada. They have been proven to be both effective and easy to use. We think you will find them to be immediately useful in your day-to-day activities.

The book is divided into three parts. Part One describes major changes in the definition and pursuit of quality in health care. Part Two focuses on the ten-step monitoring and evaluation process developed by the Joint Commission. Part Three applies the principles of quality management described in the first unit to the quality program itself.

To help the reader understand current trends in quality in health care, Chapter 1 is devoted to this topic. Chapter 2 describes THE BLUEPRINT for Quality Management and provides an overview of this organizing framework. Chapter 3 explains the shift from quality assurance to quality management. Each of the next ten chapters is devoted to a step in the Joint Commission's monitoring and evaluation process. Each chapter explains the step, interprets it in concrete terms, and suggests a practical approach to undertaking the step. Chapters 14, 15, and 16 focus on the quality program itself. Chapter 14 discusses the development of standards related to quality. Chapter 15 describes issues in evaluation and Chapter 16 examines quality improvement for the quality program itself. A clinical example of pain management is used to illustrate how the tools described in Chapters 8 through 12 fit together as a complete study.

As educators and authors, we believe that one learns best when one can relate new information to something that is already known. Also, because information about quality management can be a bit dry, we have chosen to introduce each chapter with an enlightening quote and a relevant story, anecdote, or joke. The world's greatest teachers were great storytellers. We hope that you will enjoy the levity and that the message of the stories will help you understand the thrust of the chapters.

Following the guidelines provided in this book, you will have all the elements necessary for compliance with the Joint Commission's quality assessment and improvement requirements. If you are new to quality management, the book will guide you through the process, step by step. If you already have a program in place, you can use the book as a reference to improve or streamline your current plan. Regardless of your previous experience, we think you will find tools which will help you reduce the "paper tiger" of quality management.

It was our intent as authors to provide a simple, realistic approach to developing a decentralized quality management program that would be easy for staff to "live" with, yet comprehensive enough to meet accreditation requirements. Good luck!

Jackie and Ellie

CONTENTS

Part One

DEVELOPING A FOUNDATION FOR QUALITY MANAGEMENT

1

In Pursuit of a
Definition of Quality

Styles Stipulation:
"As a word gains in popularity, it loses in clarity"
MARGRETTA M. STYLES

COSTELLO: Hey, Abbott, tell me the names of the players on our baseball team so I can say hello to them.

ABBOTT: Sure, Now, Who's on first, What's on second, I-Don't-Know on third . . .

COSTELLO: Wait a minute.

ABBOTT: What's the matter?

COSTELLO: I want to know the names of the players.

ABBOTT: I'm telling you. Who's on first, What's on second, I-Don't-Know on third . . .

COSTELLO: Now, wait. What's the name of the first baseman?

ABBOTT: No, What's the name of the second baseman.

COSTELLO: I don't know.

ABBOTT: He's the third baseman.

COSTELLO: Let's start over.

ABBOTT: Okay. Who's on first . . .

COSTELLO: I'm asking *you* what's the name of the first baseman.

ABBOTT: What's the name of the second baseman.

COSTELLO: I don't know.

ABBOTT: He's on third.

COSTELLO: All I'm trying to find out is the name of the first baseman.

ABBOTT: I keep telling you. Who's on first.

COSTELLO: I'm asking YOU what's the name of the first baseman.

ABBOTT *(Rapidly):* What's the name of the second baseman.

COSTELLO *(More rapidly):* I don't know.

BOTH *(Most rapidly):* Third base!!

COSTELLO: All right. Okay. You won't tell what's the name of the first baseman.

ABBOTT: I've *been* telling you. What's the name of the second baseman.

COSTELLO: I'm asking *you* who's on second.

ABBOTT: *Who's* on *first.*

COSTELLO: I don't know.

ABBOTT: He's on third.

COSTELLO: Let's do it this way. You pay the players on this team?

ABBOTT: Absolutely.

COSTELLO: All right. Now, when you give the first baseman his paycheck, who gets the money?

ABBOTT: Every penny of it.

COSTELLO: *Who?*
ABBOTT: Naturally.
COSTELLO: *Naturally?*
ABBOTT: Of course.
COSTELLO: All right. Than Naturally's on first . . .
ABBOTT: No. Who's on first.
COSTELLO: *I'm asking you!* What's the name of the first baseman?
ABBOTT: And I'm telling you! What's the name of the second baseman.
COSTELLO: You say third base, I'll . . . *(Pause)* Wait a minute. You got a pitcher on this team?
ABBOTT: Did you ever hear of a team without a pitcher?
COSTELLO: All right. Tell me the pitcher's name.
ABBOTT: Tomorrow.
COSTELLO: You don't want to tell me now?
ABBOTT: I said I'd tell you. Tomorrow.
COSTELLO: What's wrong with today?
ABBOTT: Nothing. He's a pretty good catcher.
COSTELLO: Who's the catcher?
ABBOTT: No, Who's the first baseman.
COSTELLO: All right, tell me that. What's the first baseman's name?
ABBOTT: No, What's the second baseman's name.
COSTELLO: I-don't-know-third-base.
ABBOTT: Look, it's very simple.
COSTELLO: I know it's simple. You got a pitcher. Tomorrow. He throws the ball to Today. Today throws the ball to Who, he throws the ball to What, What throws the ball to I-Don't-Know, *he's* on third . . . and what's more, I-Don't-Give-A-Darn!
ABBOTT: What's that?
COSTELLO: I said, I-Don't-Give-A-Darn.
ABBOTT: Oh, he's our shortstop.*

=====

The historical development of quality in health care reads somewhat like the above Abbott and Costello routine. While consumers and providers agree that quality is a major issue in health care today, nobody is quite sure "who's on first."

One of the important challenges facing health care today is to define "quality." Individual definitions are numerous, and one can easily be confused by the verbiage. Ask any nurse what is meant by the term and he or she may have difficulty putting the concept into words. Describe for that nurse a patient situation, however, and he or she can easily point out the factors that indicate quality care or the lack of it.

Quality in health care has been affected by the retrenchment that has occurred throughout American industry over the past decade. Like other businesses, health care has been harmed by the upheaval of its economic base. The combination of the Tax Equity and Fiscal Responsibility Act (TEFRA) and prospective payment has shaken the foundation of the health care industry; moreover, the nation's medical bill rose to $615 billion in 1989, a 10.8 percent increase. Higher labor costs, failure of the government's efforts to curtail costs by limiting reimbursement, and a growing number of uninsured Americans are wreaking havoc in the industry. At the same time the demand for quality services is greater than ever.

---

*This version of "Who's on First?" first appeared in *The Fireside Book of Baseball*, edited by Charles Einstein (New York, Simon & Schuster, 1956). Used with permission.

As a major American industry, health care has now begun to study the strategies used by other businesses to foster both excellence and economic survival. These methods are beginning to exert a significant effect on how the health care industry looks at quality.

■ QUALITY IN BUSINESS

Concepts of quality that are bringing about a restructuring of health care are grounded in the works of experts such as Fiegenbaum, Crosby, and Deming. The importance of quality in business first began to be appreciated in the 1940s and 1950s. Initial efforts focused primarily on the manufacturing sector; the need for quality in the service industry was later recognized.

In 1951, Fiegenbaum defined quality straightforwardly as the capability of a product to fulfill its intended purpose, produced with the least possible cost.[6] A complementary relationship between quality and cost was thus established early on.

Philip Crosby acknowledges the importance of the relationship of quality and cost but broadens the definition to include conformance to requirements; that is, quality is achieved through compliance with defined specifications or standards. Poor quality results from nonconformance. In Crosby's view, quality is not synonymous with luxury or goodness. A product or a service that conforms to its specifications demonstrates quality, whatever the product. "Quality is an achievable, measurable, profitable entity once you have commitment and understanding and are prepared for hard work."[3] Crosby emphasizes the need to do things right the first time; his concept of "zero defects" is being implemented throughout industry.

W. Edwards Deming helped the Japanese to rebuild their economy after World War II. His techniques became the standard for the Japanese; the success of Japanese business and its dominant economic position is often attributed to his influence. His strategy centers first and foremost on the development of quality and its continual improvement. The idea underlying his 14-point system is to do things right the first time, with emphasis on meeting both company and customer expectations as the primary source of quality improvement. Deming's 14 points are summarized in the box on page 6.

The Disney Company exemplifies Deming's commitment to internal and external customers in creating quality service. The Disney culture has two focal points: its customers (guests) and its employees (cast members). Guests will receive only the sort of treatment management desires provided the cast members receive the same sort of treatment. In orientation, new recruits learn to deal with fellow cast members as guests.

Meeting customer expectations of quality is defined as follows by Dr. Irving G. Synder, Jr., Vice President and Director of Research and Development for Dow Chemical USA: "This is what quality is all about: the customer's perception of excellence. And quality is our response to that perception."[21] Allen Jacobson, Chairman and CEO of 3M, agrees. The 3M company defines quality as a business management process to achieve consistent conformance to customer expectations. This philosophy is the basis for the company's total quality management (TQM) system.[15]

Deming's focus on continual improvement is evident in the Japanese concept of *Kaizen*—a continual improvement process involving everyone in a personal quest for excellence.[10] It is based on the belief that we must constantly improve and develop more efficient systems that will produce a higher quality at lower cost.[14] Continual improvement is a recurring theme in contemporary industrial definitions of quality.

DEMING'S 14 POINTS

1. Create constancy of purpose for service improvement.
2. Adopt the new philosophy.
3. Cease dependence on inspection to achieve quality.
4. End the practice of awarding business on price alone—make partners out of vendors.
5. Constantly improve every process for planning production and service.
6. Institute training and retraining on the job.
7. Institute leadership for system improvement.
8. Drive out fear.
9. Break down barriers between staff areas.
10. Eliminate slogan, exhortations, and targets for the work force.
11. Eliminate numerical quotas for the work force and numerical goals for the management.
12. Remove barriers to pride of workmanship.
13. Institute a vigorous program of education and self-improvement for everyone.
14. Put everyone to work on the transformation.

Harvard's David Garvin has summarized eight key dimensions that define quality. He suggests that rather than attempt to be "number one" in all aspects, the organization should focus on a few of these dimensions. According to Garvin, the key dimensions of quality are as follows:

- Performance or the primary operating characteristics of a service
- Features or the secondary characteristics that supplement the service's basic functioning
- Reliability or the probability of malfunction or failure within a specified period of time
- Conformance or the degree to which a service meets preestablished industry standards
- Durability or the amount of use one gets from a product before it physically deteriorates
- Serviceability or speed, courtesy, competence and ease of repair; responsiveness
- Aesthetics or how a product looks, feels, tastes, sounds, smells
- Perceived quality or what the customer thinks is quality.[8]

■ APPLYING BUSINESS CONCEPTS TO HEALTH CARE

The emphasis on quality in industry is evident in the number of theories about it. Although the primary focus of each theorist may differ, there appear to be similarities in all of the theories that have applications to health care.

The first is that quality can be defined and measured. It may be defined on the basis of specifications on the company's side and on the basis of expectations on the customer's side. These specifications take into consideration the customer's needs and wants. In applying business principles of quality to health care, certain problems have evolved. Defining quality according to customer expectations is controversial. A poll conducted for the magazine *Hospitals* revealed that a patient's satisfaction with the hospital experience represented more than half of the overall evaluation of the quality of care provided. Concern on the part of staff had the greatest influence on the patient's overall rating. While patients are capable of evaluating the quality of the hotel services provided (e.g., whether food is served at the proper temperature, and whether the staff is courteous), they are less capable of evaluating whether the correct IV fluid is dripping at the appropriate rate.[9]

The perspective of the customer is very important but it may not be as important in the health care delivery process as the measurable quality of the delivery processes that provide care during a customer's service episode.[23]

Second, quality is dynamic—it is not simply achieved and then disregarded. Quality develops from continual improvement. Tom Peters says that all quality is relative. "Each day, each product or service is getting relatively better or relatively worse, but it never stands still."[21] This is particularly true in a service business such as health care, since it is not possible to accumulate an inventory of services.

Third, quality involves a competitive edge. Philip Crosby states, "Quality is free. It's not a gift but it is free. What costs money are the unquality things—all the actions that involve not doing jobs right the first time."[3] Quality and cost go hand in hand. Quality is the primary source of cost reduction; however, the reverse of that statement is not true. Cost-reduction campaigns do not usually lead to improved quality and they usually do not result in long-term lower costs.[21]

Fourth, quality has to do with doing the "right" things right. It is estimated that poor quality accounts for 40% of the cost of people and assets in a service firm.[21] As a result, almost every other person is working on fixing something that should have already been done rather than accomplishing a new task. There is no excuse for failure to do things right the first time. Peters describes the need for quality obsession.[21] Whether or not it is possible to achieve 100% quality in a service program, if one does not strive for 100% mistakes are what one will get. Approach each patient as 100% and the variation will consist of justifiable outliers, those patients who would have ended up with a c-section or a pressure ulcer despite our best efforts rather than resulting from our mistakes. In health care, part of the answer to labor shortages may lie not in hiring more staff or developing new levels of personnel, but in refocusing efforts toward achieving zero deficits. Hospital administrators are now beginning to appreciate that a significant amount of the labor cost is related to the tremendous amount of rework that goes on.

Fifth, quality relates to outcome. The late Ray Brown, hospital administrator and past president of the American Hospital Association, said, "Doing something may be confused with getting something done."[1] The focus of all quality efforts must be on the results produced. Emphasis is on what is achieved, not solely on what is done. Management guru Peter Drucker supports this idea. "Quality in a product or service is not what a supplier puts in. It is what the customer gets out and is willing to pay for."[5] This approach also emphasizes a results orientation.

Robert Kemmel, Vice President of Corporate Marketing and Communications at Albert Einstein Health Care Foundation, states that in the year 2000 there will be 40% fewer hospitals, because of the retrenchment that will occur because of the new focus on outcomes: "Does the patient become healthier as a result of the care provided?"[11]

Sixth, quality is everyone's responsibility. Peters and Waterman advocate a strong sense of personal accountability among all employees. The attitude that each member is the company must prevail.[22] Dennis O'Leary, President of the Joint Commission on Accreditation of Health Care Organizations (Joint Commission), states that there is a long tradition of giving no more than lip service to quality. "Quality . . . is everybody's business—not simply that of the quality assurance office."[18] Commitment must be made at the executive level and permeate the organization. It must be at the top of everyone's agenda, foremost in everyone's mind. As the current Ford Motor Company slogan puts it, "Quality is job one."

■ DEFINITIONS OF QUALITY IN HEALTH CARE

Definitions of quality in health care tend to focus on the technical aspects of quality. The National Association of Quality Assurance Professionals describes quality as levels of excellence produced and documented in the process of patient care based on the best knowledge available and achievable at a particular facility.[12]

The Joint Commission defines quality as "the degree to which patient care services increase the probability of desired outcomes and reduce the probability of undesired outcomes given the current state of knowledge."[7] With the Joint Commission's Agenda for Change, the emphasis on defining quality has shifted from quality as a process-oriented variable to quality results or outcomes. The Joint Commission has recently outlined 12 factors that determine the quality of patient care. These factors and their definitions appear in the box on page 9.

Differences among institutions regarding factors contributing to quality were shown in a survey done among 663 CEOs. In hospitals with more than 400 beds, the medical staff tended to be ranked as most significant; while in hospitals with 200 to 400 beds, the nursing staff was more likely to be ranked as most significant. Overall, nursing care was mentioned as one of the three most significant factors in 97.3% of the responses. Clinical skills of the medical staff ranked second (96.4%) and employee attitudes ranked third (93.3%).[13]

The pursuit of an all-embracing definition of quality has been elusive. Donabedian suggests that no one definition will suffice, and proposes three definitions: (1) the *absolutist* definition considers the possibility of benefit and harm to health as valued by the practitioner, with no attention to cost; (2) the *individualized* definition focuses on the patient's expectations of benefit and/or harm and other undesired consequences; and (3) the *social* definition includes the cost of care, the benefit/harm continuum, and the distribution of health care as valued by the population in general.[4] C. Duane Dauner, President of the California Hospital Association, states, "It can no longer simply be defined by what technology is available. The challenge facing providers is to balance human values, technological resources, quality of life and innovation with economic reality, to provide the best possible care."[16]

It does not appear that a universal definition of quality is forthcoming. Nevertheless, even in the absence of a formal definition, a patient or provider can certainly identify its absence—substandard care or less-than-optimal results. Three or more attempts at venipuncture, or serving hot meals cold exemplify substandard care. Pressure ulcers and postoperative infections are examples of poor outcomes.

■ STANDARDS DEFINE QUALITY

The quality of care which is expected from a health care facility is made explicit by written standards that direct the way the service is to be provided and the results that should be achieved from that service. Standards, therefore, define quality.

A standard is a written value statement of rules, conditions, and actions in a patient, staff member, or the system that are sanctioned by an appropriate authority. There are four components to this definition.

The first is that the standard is written. Holding staff accountable for unwritten

---

FACTORS THAT DETERMINE QUALITY OF PATIENT CARE

Accessibility to care: the ease with which a patient can obtain the care he/she needs.

Timeliness of care: the degree to which care is made available to a patient when it is needed.

Effectiveness of care: the degree to which the care rendered is provided in the correct manner, given the current state of the art.

Efficacy of care: the degree to which a service has the potential to meet the need for which it is used.

Appropriateness of care: the degree to which the care received matches the needs of the patient.

Efficiency of care: the degree to which the care received has the desired effect with a minimum of possible effort, expense, or waste.

Continuity of care: the degree to which the care needed by the patient is coordinated effectively among practitioners and across organizations and time.

Privacy of care: the rights of a patient to control the distribution and release of data concerning his/her illness, including information provided to health care professionals and any additional information contained in the medical record and/or other source documents.

Confidentiality of care: information the health care team obtains from or about a patient that is considered to be privileged and thus, except in specified circumstances, that may vary by illness and jurisdiction, cannot be disclosed to a third party without the patient's consent.

Participation of patient and patient family in care: patient (or patient family) involvement in the decision-making process in matters pertaining to his/her health.

Safety of care environment: the degree to which necessary spaces, equipment, and medications are available to the patient when needed.

Copyright 1989 by the Joint Commission on Accreditation of Healthcare Organizations, Oakbrook Terrace, IL. Reprinted from Quality Review Bulletin 15(11):331, with permission.

or word-of-mouth standards is like trying to pin Jell-O to the wall . . . virtually impossible! The standards adhere to current acceptable levels of practice, and are presented in a form that is easily understood by those who are expected to conform to them.

Secondly, standards define a set of rules, actions, or conditions. Rules constitute the structure of the service, actions are the process of how the service is carried out, and conditions define the results or outcomes of the services. Structure standards define the rules under which the service must be delivered, for example, all patients transported by wheelchair or gurney must have a seat belt in place. Structure standards are nonnegotiable and nonmodifiable.

Process standards define how the service is to be carried out. Examples of process standards include the procedures, protocols, and care plans that direct service delivery. Process standards are modifiable based on the individual practitioner's analysis of the situation at hand. For example, a process standard might suggest that peripheral IV sites be rotated every 72 hours. On assessment of Mrs. Jones, an 85-year-old patient with inadequate veins, the nurse determines that her IV is patent and there are no signs of phlebitis or infection after 3 days; weighing these facts, the nurse decides not to rotate the IV site but rather to maintain the current site and monitor it closely.

Outcome standards define both the desired results to be achieved and the undesirable results to be avoided. They are part and parcel of every process standard. The service provided must lead to a clearly defined and measurable outcome. Process and outcomes are inseparable.

The third critical component is that standards are written for patients, staff, and systems. Quality must permeate the organization. Standards must state what patients are to receive, how staff are to function, and how the system is to operate. These three components are integrally linked. The finest clinical standards will not facilitate quality if staff are not competent to carry them out, or if there are not enough staff to comply.

Finally, the standard must be approved by an authority. An authority is a group or individual empowered to enforce the standard and to hold staff accountable. Without proper sanctioning the standard may be ignored. There are many sources of sanctioning. Hierarchical approval is the most common; however, a significant and powerful source of sanctioning comes from the individuals who are expected to uphold the standard in their day-to-day practice. The endorsement and support of staff are critical to both implementation and monitoring of standards. Compliance with standards is more likely if those involved feel that they are achievable and especially if it is a standard they played a role in setting.

■ DEFINING QUALITY ASSURANCE

Philip Crosby states that "quality is free but no one is ever going to know it if there isn't some sort of agreed-on system of measurement."[3] Smeltzer defines quality assurance (QA) as the systematic testing and evaluation of nursing practice.[24]

The position of the American Nurses' Association (ANA) is that QA is the sum of all the activities that ensure that patients receive the best possible nursing care. It focuses on solving problems and measuring achievement of standards.[17] Norma Lang states, "In the broadest sense QA is both a concomitant and an outgrowth of what all of us are going through in our society at large: an attempt to define who we are, how we relate to one another, how we feel about issues, how we come to grips with our values, and how we can act most responsibly on those values."[17]

Coyne and Killien describe QA as a process directed toward evaluating patient care that is provided in a particular setting through developing standards for care and implementing mechanisms for ensuring that the standards are met.[2]

According to the Joint Commission, QA is the process for objectively and systematically monitoring and evaluating the quality and appropriateness of patient care, for pursuing opportunities to improve patient care, and for resolving identified problems.[7] Appropriateness refers to the extent to which a particular procedure or treatment is efficacious, is clearly indicated, is neither excessive nor deficient, and is provided in a setting best suited to the patient's needs.[20]

■ OUR DEFINITION OF QUALITY ASSURANCE

Quality assurance is a process, not an episode. It is an orderly series of activities designed to corroborate the defined attributes of quality. It is the process of ensuring conformance with requirements, that is, that staff are in compliance with the written standards. In other words, it is the process of ensuring that what was specified actually occurs, that things turn out as intended—every time.

Quality assurance is a means, not an end. It is the process of guaranteeing quality. Traditionally, that has meant identifying and resolving problems; today it means guaranteeing the quality of process and outcomes. Traditionally it has meant *controlling* the level of quality within an organization; today it means *managing* the quality provided with a focus on continual improvement. As Dennis O'Leary so aptly states, "Even if it ain't broke, it can still be improved."[19] Consider the strides that have been made on Alexander Graham Bell's great invention, the telephone!

Trudy, the bag lady in Jane Wagner's *The Search for Signs of Intelligent Life in the Universe,* states, "I worry whoever thought up the term 'quality control' thought if we didn't control it, it would get out of hand."[25]

Traditionally, quality assurance has been defined as the process of setting standards, monitoring practice, evaluating practice problems, and resolving practice problems. Future perspectives on quality shift the emphasis from problem identification to problem prevention, from assurance to management. This new approach to managing quality in health care stems from the knowledge that quality is the competitive edge.

In order to guarantee quality through preventive efforts, there must be a way to measure the quality of the service provided and the outcomes achieved.

■ HOW DO WE MEASURE QUALITY?

The first step in assessing quality is to define it through clear written standards. Once this has been accomplished, the fit between what is supposed to be done and what actually occurs can be evaluated. Analysis of conformance to written standards is the benchmark by which quality is measured.

Assessment is systematic and continuous. It is done in an orderly fashion over time, not as a single event. It must occur at the point of contact with the customer and should be carried out by those who are delivering the service. It must be done *by* the work group not *to* them.

In health care, the most widely accepted format for assessing quality is the 10-step monitoring and evaluation process outlined by the Joint Commission.

Monitoring is defined as the planned, systematic, and ongoing collection, compilation, and organization of data about an indicator of the quality and/or appropriateness of an important aspect of care, and the comparison of those data to an established level of performance (threshold for evaluation) to determine the need for in-depth evaluation. Evaluation is that assessment activity related to determining the meaning and importance of the data collected. It includes making judgments about both the quality and the appropriateness of nursing care based on comparisons between the observed practices of the nursing service and the predetermined, well-defined clinical indicator.[20]

The 10 steps of the monitoring and evaluation model are as follows:

1. Assign responsibility.
2. Delineate the scope of care and service.
3. Identify important aspects of care and service.
4. Identify indicators.
5. Establish thresholds for evaluation.
6. Collect and organize data.
7. Evaluate.
8. Take action.
9. Assess actions and document improvement.
10. Communicate relevant information.

The Joint Commission lists eight essential characteristics of effective monitoring and evaluation activities:

- Are planned, systematic, and ongoing
- Are comprehensive
- Use "indicators" and related thresholds agreed on by the department/service staff and acceptable to the organization

- Are accomplished by the routine collection of data related to the indicators and periodic comparison of the level of performance with thresholds for evaluations
- Include evaluation of important aspects of care when the thresholds for evaluation are reached
- Result in appropriate actions to solve identified problems or to take other identified opportunities to improve patient care
- Are continual in an effort to ensure sustained improvements in care and performance
- Are integrated with other services and merged, as appropriate, with information obtained throughout the organization

A successful monitoring and evaluation process is ongoing and integrated into every aspect of the services it is designed to measure. The monitoring and evaluation process takes place within the context of the nursing department as a whole. Nursing has a mechanism for coordinating, facilitating, and integrating the monitoring and evaluation process throughout the division. There is a master plan that enables nursing management to maximize its investment in monitoring the services it provides and the results of those services. THE BLUEPRINT for Quality Management, which will be described in Chapter 2, is one such organizing framework.

REFERENCES

1. Brownisms: Words of wisdom on management style, Hospitals, p 88, December 5, 1989.
2. Coyne C and Killien M: A system for unit-based monitors of quality of nursing care, J Nurs Admin 17(1):26-32, July-August 1983.
3. Crosby PB: Quality is free, New York, 1979, New American Library.
4. Donabedian A: Explorations in quality assessment and monitoring, vol II: The criteria and standards of quality, Ann Arbor, 1982, Health Administration Press.
5. Drucker PI: Innovation and entrepreneurship, New York, 1985, Harper & Row Publishers.
6. Fiegenbaum AV: Quality control, New York, 1951, McGraw-Hill Book Company.
7. Fromberg R, editor: Monitoring and evaluation in nursing services, 1986, Joint Commission on Accreditation of Hospitals.
8. Garvin DA: Competing on the eight dimensions of quality, Harvard Bus Rev, pp 101-109, Nov/Dec 1987.
9. How consumers perceive health care quality, Hospitals, p 84, April 5, 1988.
10. Kerfoot K and Rohe D: KAIZEN: innovations for nurse managers to improve productivity, Nurs Econ 7(4):228-230, July-August 1989.
11. Kemmel RB: Agreeing on a definition of quality care may be healthcare's biggest challenge, Modern Healthcare, p 37, March 24, 1989.
12. Kibbie PE, editor: Quality assurance, utilization and risk management: A study guide, 1986, National Association of Quality Assurance Professionals.
13. Koska M: Quality—thy name is nursing care, CEOs say, Hospitals, p 32, February 5, 1989.
14. Masaaki I: KAIZEN: The key to Japan's competitive success, New York, 1986, Random House.
15. Melum M and Siniores M: The next generation of health care quality, Hospitals, p 80, February 5, 1989.
16. NEWS: California Hospital Association, Sacramento, 18(21), September 12, 1986.
17. Nursing Quality Assurance Management/Learning System, Missouri, 1982, American Nurses' Association and California Suterland Learning Associates.
18. O'Leary D: President's column, Joint Comm Perspect 8(1/2):2-3, January/February, 1988.
19. O'Leary D and Ripple H: Responding to harsh criticism of the JCAHO, Nurs Econ 7(3):126-128, May-June, 1989.
20. Patterson CH: Standards of patient care: the Joint Commission's focus on nursing quality assurance, Nurs Clin North Am 23(3):625-637, September 1988.
21. Peters T: Thriving on chaos, New York, 1988, Knopf.
22. Peters T and Waterman R: In search of excellence, New York, 1982, Harper & Row Publishers.
23. Productivity and performance management in health care institutions, 1989, American Hospital Publishing, Inc.
24. Smeltzer CH, Henshaw AS, and Feltman B: The benefits of staff nurse involvement in monitoring the quality of patient care, J Nurs Qual Assur 3:1-7, 1987.
25. Wagner J: The search for signs of intelligent life in the universe, New York, 1986, Harper & Row Publishers.

2

THE BLUEPRINT FOR QUALITY MANAGEMENT

If you always do what you've always done,
you'll always get what you've always gotten.
JAY KATZ

■ NEEDED: CREATIVITY IN QA

The 1949 movie "The Fountainhead," based on the novel by Ayn Rand, portrays architects as a group of noncreative technicians who design buildings with little thought and imagination. The film shows students in a school of architecture receiving accolades for creating blueprints that clone the world's existing structures. Only one student, Howard Roark, creates bold, innovative designs. His teachers do not recognize his talent and reject his work. Unfazed by rejection, Roark continues creating magnificent structures that deviate from the accepted standard. Architectural experts label him a rebellious renegade and place little value on his work. The climax of the story occurs when Howard Roark agrees to design, in secret and free of charge, a low-income housing project. He receives a promise that the project will be built *exactly* as designed, without changes or modifications.

As the project proceeds the experts incorporate their preconceived notions of building design into the structure. They are uncomfortable with the housing project until its design matches the surrounding buildings.

Appalled and embarrassed by the finished construction, Roark reduces the monstrosity to a heap of rubble in a spectacular dynamite blast. The movie concludes with Roark's arrest and dramatic trial in which he successfully defends his actions.

This story could just as easily be scripted about quality assurance in health care today. The architectural "experts" of 1949 were comfortable with cumbersome, inefficient designs for buildings. They were hesitant to incorporate new ideas that deviated from the accepted standard. Many of today's health care organizations also are comfortable with cumbersome, inefficient designs of quality assurance methodology. They also are hesitant to incorporate new ideas that deviate from accepted QA standards.

For years many health care organizations viewed QA as a fixed process. Accreditation requirements tended to stifle creativity and experimentation. Fear of appearing "wrong" in the eyes of QA "experts" and failing the accreditation process was very real. Attempts to change or improve a system were often hesitantly, fearfully, and quietly undertaken, or squashed altogether.

Unfortunately, the traditional QA mind set is difficult to change. We are creatures of habit. Roger von Oech in *A Whack on the Side of the Head* illustrates this "creature of habit" phenomenon in a simple exercise that shows how quickly and unwittingly a "mind set" can develop.[7] This exercise demonstrates how easily our minds "lock in" to a point of view. Here is the exercise. See if your mind quickly "locks in," too.

Shown below is Roman numeral 9. By adding only a single line, turn it into a 6.

IX

Did you find yourself struggling to turn this Roman numeral into a 6? It takes a creative thinker to solve this puzzle. Creative thinkers are able to think "out of context." Consider the IX not as Roman numerals, but rather as letters in the English language. Now add a single line, in the shape of an "S" preceding the "IX." The result is six. Many people are unable to step out of context to solve this puzzle. With only one example of a Roman numeral—IX—they are locked into the context of Roman numerals.

Solving a problem like the one described above requires creative thinking. Likewise, today's health care industry faces monumental problems that require creative thinking for solutions. However, it will be very difficult to find solutions if the health care industry is locked into a traditional QA mind set and is unable to step out of context for solutions. "We've never done it that way before" must not become the basis for decision making.

As any observer of today's health care system can attest, standards, quality assessment, and improvement are the focus of an industry-wide revolution. There is a search for creative solutions to the problems facing health care. Every aspect of care, practice, and governance must, of necessity, come under scrutiny. Human and monetary resources are no longer available for inefficient health care, ineffective management, and meaningless quality assurance. Finding new ways to deliver more efficient and less costly health care is mandatory for the industry's survival. In large measure this survival will depend on the industry's willingness to develop more effective quality management practices.

■ THE BLUEPRINT FOR QUALITY MANAGEMENT: A CREATIVE MANAGEMENT PLAN

THE BLUEPRINT for Quality Management is a creative, comprehensive quality management plan designed for the division of nursing. The name, THE BLUEPRINT, originated from a consideration of the model's attributes and its unique, comprehensive design, or blueprint. Blueprint is a term used in the construction industry. It denotes not only thought and creativity but also construction and accomplishment. Just as Howard Roark, the architect of "The Fountainhead," used his blueprints to guide the construction of unique buildings, so THE BLUEPRINT guides the construction of a unique division-wide quality management program.

THE BLUEPRINT differs from *all* other models by expanding beyond clinical practice. In the past, models focused on direct patient care given by the nurse. Now, for the first time, a model exists to organize and manage not just patient care, but an entire division of nursing.

This model dispels the old notion that nursing consists *exclusively* of direct patient care—clinical practice—and therefore only direct patient care should be monitored. THE BLUEPRINT reflects the reality that every patient is the recipient of services from three distinct domains of practice: clinical, professional, and administrative. This model is then used to direct monitoring and evaluation in each domain.

The idea of monitoring each domain to solve the problems within health care is innovative and unique to THE BLUEPRINT. For years the narrow focus of QA in the health care industry has plagued conscientious nurses. Dennis O'Leary, President of the Joint Commission, put it well in a May 14, 1990 speech to the American Organization of Nurse Executives in Baltimore, Maryland when he said, "Most problems in health care today are systems problems and staff are victims of the system."[5]

A good example of the truth of O'Leary's statement occurred recently in a large medical center. The infection control department discovered a sudden, dramatic increase in urinary tract infections in catheterized patients. Alarmed, the administration devoted time, money, and staff to remedying the "poor nursing care." After weeks of investigation of their nursing staff, someone thought to culture the "sterile" Foley catheters. The catheters were found to be contaminated. This organization is to be commended for finding the source of the infection. However, weeks of distress among the nursing staff could have been avoided had each domain been looked into in the first place.

When THE BLUEPRINT is operationalized within an organization, every problem is viewed from a trifocus: clinical, professional, and administrative. Each problem is addressed by asking what part the patient, the staff, and the system contributes. The framework requires health care professionals to analyze every problem from this triple perspective. The flow chart in Figure 2-1 illustrates the problem-solving process using THE BLUEPRINT.

The key to understanding today's QA focus is to consider nursing care not as a series of tasks, but as a collection of results. Many factors affect results. Very rarely are either positive or negative outcomes the result of actions of one single health care provider. What happens to a patient within a health care organization may be the result of the patient's actions, the staff's actions, the system's actions, or a combination of the three. Monitoring only the functions of the nursing staff creates a narrow focus. When monitoring focuses exclusively on the nurse's actions, problems created by other members of the health care team or the organization may be missed or go uncorrected. A goal of the organization is positive and appropriate individual patient outcomes. No segment of health care stands alone. All are interdependent. Achievement of positive patient outcomes can occur only through a *team effort* of health care workers in concert with a supportive *system*. Likewise, monitoring needs a team or global focus.

This global focus was perceived and illustrated by Donabedian in the 1960s and conceptually diagrammed as a cube that portrayed the type of variables, the level of

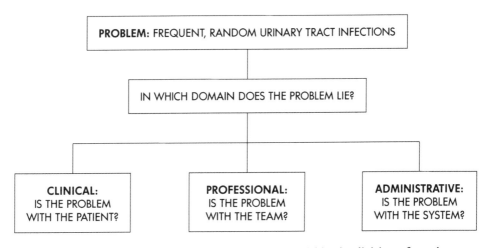

■ **FIGURE 2-1**   **Flowchart for problem solving within the division of nursing.**

analysis, and the scope of analysis.[2] The cube was adapted in 1976 by the American Nurses' Association.[1] The concept integrated structure, process, and outcome with the patient, nursing, and the nursing organization, but the concept remained undeveloped as a concrete, practical, usable framework until development of THE BLUEPRINT.

Quality management requires new and creative methods for evaluation. It provides an opportunity to reevaluate long-standing monitoring and evaluation methods. Process-oriented monitoring, focusing on what the nurse does, is replaced by outcome-oriented monitoring that evaluates patient outcomes from all three domains.

This philosophy also renders many earlier quality assurance practices obsolete. "Volume indicators," for example, which was a collection of data describing how much, how many, and how often is now of little value except to establish baseline data for setting thresholds. "Volumes" such as how many falls, how many medication errors, and so on, have little impact on improvement within the organization. Merely collecting data is comparable to a sports announcer saying, "Good evening, ladies and gentlemen. Last night's football scores were 7-9, 21-7, a tie, and 17-14 in overtime." The station would be inundated with callers wanting to know who had scored, where, and how. In other words, scores alone are meaningless. Although the score or outcome is the visible, reportable result, what led to it is a complicated process. To report "volumes" like "how many" or "how much" without analysis and without an action plan for improvement is of no benefit and a waste of resources.

The new quality management philosophy incorporated in THE BLUEPRINT redirects the previous emphasis on tasks. In the past, health care professionals placed great emphasis on procedural issues and correctly performed tasks. It was very important that each nurse follow every step of the procedure. Checklists of tasks served as a popular monitoring tool. This method gave rise to a much-quoted, tongue-in-cheek quip, "The procedure was perfect, but the patient died," for the emphasis was not on patient outcome, but on performance of nursing tasks. While nursing tasks performed correctly are important, they are not the goal of quality management. The correct "by-the-textbook" insertion of a Foley catheter by a rude, grumpy employee is *still* unacceptable care. Providing a checklist of skills validating this employee's competency will not convince the patient that he or she received quality care.

■ THE BLUEPRINT INCORPORATES THREE SYSTEMS OF QUALITY MANAGEMENT

THE BLUEPRINT offers a commonsense approach to quality management. It incorporates not only the three domains mentioned earlier, but also the three systems necessary to a successful quality management program as described by Coyne and Killien[3]: (1) a value system, (2) an appraisal or assessment system, and (3) a response system (Figure 2-2).

A value system involves *quality awareness*. The development of a value system based on written standards is the foundation of the quality management program. Standards are nothing more than the division of nursing's values expressed in writing.

Consider this conversation between two nurses in an intermediate care department.

NURSE 1: My patient has a blood glucose level of 55 on the Accu check and he is lethargic. I'm calling the lab to come and do a stat blood glucose level!

NURSE 2: Why not give him a glass of orange juice and recheck it in 5 minutes by Accu check?

NURSE 1: Because that's not the way we do it here.

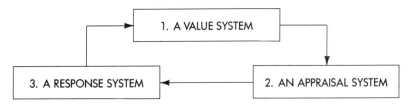

■ **FIGURE 2-2** **Three components of quality management model.**

NURSE 2: Why not?
NURSE 1: I don't know. I've been working here for 3 years and this is how we do it.
NURSE 2: Where is the practice guideline for the management of the diabetic patient? I'd like to read it.
NURSE 1: I've never heard of a practice guideline. Just trust me; this is how we do it here.

It would be difficult to develop a quality management program in this intermediate care department under their present system. Their standards are vague, implied, and conveyed by word of mouth. Standards should be *written,* in order to create a meaningful quality management program. The department described above needed a coordinated care path for the diabetic patient with accompanying practice guidelines. Practice guidelines are one of the values, or standards, of THE BLUEPRINT. Practice guidelines standardize care and govern practitioner response to a problem. They then become the basis for monitoring, the benchmarks against which conformance to requirements is measured.

Practice guidelines are only one kind of standard incorporated in THE BLUEPRINT. Standards are the foundation of THE BLUEPRINT and several formats for articulating and writing standards are used in this model. Written standards facilitate the quantitative measurement of quality. It is impossible to develop a meaningful QM program when standards are vague and implied whereas with written, organized standards quality assessment is easy to accomplish and quality improvement is measurable.

An appraisal or assessment system is synonymous with *quality assurance.* This system consists of specific evaluation activities that determine conformance to the written standards or values of the division of nursing. THE BLUEPRINT specifies not only appropriate quality assessment activities but also the methodology for carrying out those activities in an organized, predetermined manner.

THE BLUEPRINT incorporates an appraisal system in harmony with the Joint Commission's 10-step process. The tools of THE BLUEPRINT are used to carry out each step. With the aid of the tools, even a novice can create an effective monitoring and evaluation program. This second system, the appraisal system, also is necessary to a successful quality management program.

A response system involves *quality improvement.* Quality improvement is the result of a well-organized response system. A well-organized response system has appropriate action-planning mechanisms in place which can be implemented when an opportunity for improvement occurs. THE BLUEPRINT incorporates action-planning formats that enable the division of nursing to track the quality improvement process and document when and where improvement occurred.

Types of action planning included in THE BLUEPRINT are:

1. A clinical action plan: patient care plan or patient teaching plan
2. An employee development plan
3. A staff development plan
4. An administrative action plan

These plans are an integral part of THE BLUEPRINT. They are the mechanisms that demonstrate that change or improvement has occurred in response to a problem or need.

All three systems are *vitally* important to a successful quality management program and therefore carry equal weight in THE BLUEPRINT. It is impossible to design an appraisal system (QA program) apart from the value system (standards) and generate a positive response system (quality improvement) within the division of nursing unless all three systems are present and given equal attention. When the three systems of this quality management model are present, written standards will be in place, quality assessment data will be derived directly from those written standards, and quality improvement will be measurable.

■ WHY USE THE BLUEPRINT?

It is almost impossible to incorporate the three components of quality management into a division of nursing in the absence of a model. The model is the organizational plan. When the plan is in place everyone within the organization knows what is going on. In the words of Dennis O'Leary, everyone is "singing from the same hymnal."[5]

Today's nursing environment requires a model with breadth and flexibility that can fit the present and encompass the future. Models that focus attention only on patient care delivery are simply inadequate in today's high-risk, high-litigation, cost-containment, nursing-shortage environment. While various clinical practice models to monitor bedside care have been available for years, until the development of THE BLUEPRINT there were none that met multifaceted, division-wide needs.

■ HOW THE BLUEPRINT DIFFERS FROM OTHER MODELS

THE BLUEPRINT differs from other models in that it contains far more than a theoretical, clinical practice framework. THE BLUEPRINT emphasizes division-wide standards. An accompanying quality assessment program and organized response mechanisms also are part of THE BLUEPRINT.

This division-wide approach to standards development, quality assessment and improvement, makes it practical and functional. Yet, it is flexible enough to be used in any division of nursing regardless of an individual health care facility's philosophy, goals, or organizational structure.

■ THE BLUEPRINT IS USER FRIENDLY

THE BLUEPRINT eliminates concern and confusion by not only providing concrete mechanisms and formats for developing nursing standards, but also by detailing formats and methodology for monitoring, evaluating, and improving them. It is a clinically tested, reality-based model that serves as the division of nursing's master plan for organizing, standardizing, monitoring, evaluating, and improving every aspect of care, practice, and governance within the division of nursing.

■ BACKGROUND OF THE BLUEPRINT

THE BLUEPRINT grew out of the chaos created in the U.S. health care system during the past decade. As health care costs spiraled, as the government sought to contain costs through prospective payment, and as the nursing shortage altered health care delivery, existing mechanisms to control quality became inadequate. Evolution of the Joint Commission's mission, standards, requirements, and accreditation methodology, while praiseworthy, nevertheless are contributing to the chaos. As each new regulatory body announces changes in requirements and new terminology, nurses are becoming increasingly baffled by the dilemma posed of keeping up with the terminology and changing requirements. With fewer employees, fewer resources, and more critically ill patients, many nurses' perceptions of QA became skewed. As one nurse put it, "I'm spending valuable time away from patient care on meaningless QA." Like this nurse, many health care professionals charged with responsibility for quality assurance are becoming frustrated in their efforts to distinguish between "important" and "waste of time" monitoring. There is the added question of who controls and acts on the collected data.

The increased health care litigation of the 1980s produced a flurry of QA activities. These activities, carried out vigorously in a variety of experimental and costly ways by sincere and dedicated professionals, received little commitment or understanding from members of the organizational hierarchies. For many chief executive officers, quality assurance activities were mandatory for accreditation but otherwise were of little or no value.

Convinced that quality assurance was not a board level function, many administrators pointed to the flurry of QA activity and were satisfied that their institutions practiced "quality." They were certain that their QA program was exceptional, for, after all, they received accreditation, and they viewed accreditation as an indication of success. Yet true success is the demonstration of excellence in patient care delivery—not just a paper score from an accrediting body.

This philosophy, that true success is demonstrated in excellence in patient care delivery, gave birth to THE BLUEPRINT. The 5-year period of researching and developing this model focused primarily upon *proving* excellence in patient care—and meeting accreditation requirements in the process! THE BLUEPRINT stands today as a unique system that has revolutionized conventional QA concepts because its primary goal is not *accreditation* but *excellence* in patient care delivery.

■ EXPLANATION OF THE BLUEPRINT

What is quality? How is it measured? How is the safety, effectiveness, and appropriateness of patient care delivery demonstrated? Where is an institution's proof that things happen the way they are planned to happen? THE BLUEPRINT provides mechanisms for answering these questions. It is predicated on the belief that the quality of health care is explicit in written standards and that these standards direct the delivery of nursing's services.

Viewing nursing as a service business is difficult for many nurses. The word "business" implies cost control and money management. Many nurses resist the notion. As they devote themselves to patient care, they believe an emphasis on cost in some way breaches their professional code of behavior. They believe cost to be an unimportant issue when compared to human life.

As cost containment efforts escalated, many of these professionals were forced to accept that health care organizations can no longer afford to provide *all* services to *all* patients *all* the time by *all* staff. For the first time, nurses began to view the division of nursing as a cost center and to regard their services as a business. The evolution of this new thinking has led many nurses to realize the importance of reimbursement for the profession. Reimbursement for nursing services may become a reality when nurses are able to itemize the services that they provide. While billing for nurses' services may be

THE BLUEPRINT FOR QUALITY MANAGEMENT

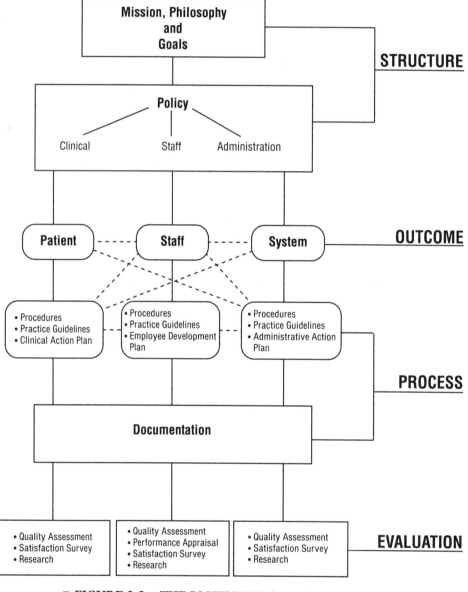

■ FIGURE 2-3   THE BLUEPRINT for quality management.

a future practice, nevertheless, nursing care should be defined in standards today. As these standards direct the distribution of nursing's time and efforts, so too will they serve as a basis for defining reimbursement of those services.

Nurses can take control of the business of nursing by developing written standards, monitoring compliance to those standards, and evaluating and improving the results. THE BLUEPRINT is designed to guide nurses in this process.

A unique feature of THE BLUEPRINT (Figure 2-3) is its organization of the division of nursing as a service business. This concept permeates the entire model. For example, in the delivery of nursing care there are always three business constants:

1. Someone who needs the service
2. Someone who delivers the service
3. Someone who manages the service

Using these constants as a basis for the model, THE BLUEPRINT is now divided into three domains:

1. A clinical domain—referring to the patient
2. A professional domain—referring to the staff
3. An administrative domain—referring to management

These domains stem directly from the business constants.

THE BLUEPRINT integrates the three domains of nursing practice with the three service areas of business. In Figure 2-3, the first vertical track represents the clinical domain. The middle or second track represents the professional domain. The third track represents the administrative domain. Clearly delineating each domain—clinical, professional, and administrative—has distinct advantages for the division of nursing. First, appropriate standards may now be written specifically for each domain. This brings organization and direction to standards development. Second, quality assessment activities may now be directed toward the identified domain to pinpoint problems or identify specific opportunities for improvement. Quality, then, will be defined by writing what is to be done in each domain, under what circumstances, and by whom. Then, by monitoring outcomes in each domain, the division of nursing measures the degree to which things are happening the way they were designed to happen.

Using this model ensures that monitoring and evaluation activities will focus not only on patient care or clinical services, but on professional and administrative services as well. Although often overlooked, the health care team and governance of the organization have a direct impact on patient care. For this reason, they must be included in the monitoring and evaluation process. Therefore, standards must be clearly defined and written in each domain. The division of nursing will then have clinical standards (dealing with patient care activities), professional standards (dealing with professional activities), and administrative standards (dealing with governance activities). Recognizing the three domains permits quality management professionals, for the first time, to understand and use three types of standards:

1. Standards of care
2. Standards of practice
3. Standards of governance

These standards translate the division of nursing's values into actions and results and define, in writing, those activities and outcomes for which staff and nursing

EXCELLENCE IN SERVICE

We believe . . .

- that each of our patients, regardless of circumstances, possess intrinsic value from God and should be treated with dignity and respect.

- that each encounter with patients and families should portray compassion and concern.

- that each patient should receive quality care that is cost-effective, competitive and based on the latest technology.

- that patient confidentiality and privacy should be preserved.

- that meeting the needs of patients and other customers should always be our number one priority.

EXCELLENCE IN PRACTICE

We believe . . .

- that our profession is a science and an art, the essence of which is nurturing and caring.

- that our primary duty is to restore and maintain the health of our patients in a spirit of compassion and concern.

- that the nursing process is an integral part of our practice as professional nurses.

- that nurses should collaborate with other health care team members to meet the holistic needs of our patients, which include physical, psychosocial and spiritual aspects of care.

- that we should aggressively promote patient and family education to allow each individual the opportunity to prevent illness and/or achieve optimal health.

- that we are accountable to our patients, patients' families and to each other for our professional practice.

- that monitoring and evaluating nursing practice is our responsibility and is necessary to continuously improve care.

- that we should pursue professional growth and development through education, participation in professional organizations and support of research.

EXCELLENCE IN LEADERSHIP

We believe . . .

- that we should provide a progressive environment, utilizing current technology, guided by responsible stewardship to promote the highest quality patient care and employee satisfaction.

- that we should encourage and support collaborative decision-making by those who are closest to the situation, even at the risk of failure.

- that compassion should be characterized in our day to day personal interactions as well as being a motivating factor in management decisions.

- that we should be sensitive to individual needs and give support, praise, and recognition to encourage professional and personal development.

- that we should possess an energy level and personal style that empowers and inspires enthusiasm in others.

- that we should consider suggestions and criticisms as challenges for improvement and innovation.

- that justice should be applied equitably in all employment practices and personnel policies.

■ FIGURE 2-4   Philosophy written in three domains. (From Memorial Hospital, Chattanooga, Tenn. Used with permission.)

management will be held accountable. Standards of care delineate the clinical domain, standards of practice delineate the professional domain, and standards of governance delineate the administrative domain. Figure 2-3 is divided horizontally into four sections to reflect the four broad-based categories of standards: structure, outcome, process, and evaluation.

Structure

Structure refers to standards that describe the rules of the system and its governance. Structure standards include mission, philosophy, goals, and policies. (THE BLUEPRINT places job descriptions in a subheading under policies because they are governance issues and are nonnegotiable.) The mission statement addresses the overall business of the division of nursing and is in harmony with the mission of the institution. The philosophy, delineating values and beliefs, is divided into three domains: clinical, professional, and administrative. The clinical practice philosophy states the division of nursing's beliefs about delivery of patient care. The professional practice philosophy states the beliefs about professional practice in the facility, and the administrative practice philosophy states the beliefs about the governance of the division of nursing. Figure 2-4 illustrates philosophy written in the three domains as developed at Memorial Hospital in Chattanooga, Tennessee.

Goals are long-range statements of purpose. They also should be written for each domain. Goals should be established for clinical practice, professional practice, and administrative practice.

The mission, philosophy, and goals of the division of nursing are important structure standards, for it is with them that the quality commitment of the organization begins.

Policies, a highly critical component of structure, also must be written for the three domains. Policies are rules and are not negotiable. They may *not* be modified under any circumstances. By writing policies for each domain and restricting them to nonnegotiable rules, an organized, concise, user-friendly policy manual emerges.

A word of caution is in order. Many divisions of nursing call every wish or rule a "policy." This is confusing to the staff. Policy is *nonnegotiable*. In a court of law an institution is bound by its policies. For this reason policies must be limited to those rules that are truly nonnegotiable. Negotiable issues are detailed in practice guidelines. Practice guidelines are negotiable; they may be modified when necessary. For example, the timing of changing IV tubing and rotating IV sites may be negotiated or altered by patient condition. These guidelines are negotiable. However, the written statement about personnel permitted to insert an IV within the institution is policy because it is nonnegotiable. For example, a nurse could not say to an LPN, "I'm busy, please go and start this IV for me," if the institution's policy states that only RNs and MDs may start IVs.

Outcome

Outcome standards never stand alone. It helps to think of outcomes as "piggy-back standards" for they are attached to all process standards. They are always the objective of another standard. In the clinical domain they are written on patient care plans, teaching plans, and clinical practice guidelines. In the professional domain they are written on employee development plans and professional practice guidelines. In the administrative domain they are written on administrative action plans and on administrative practice guidelines.

Process

Process standards are "working" standards. They describe what nurses do, what patients receive, and how the system operates. These standards address all activities of patient, staff, and system. This category includes activities such as patient care plans, practice guidelines, procedures, teaching plans, employee development plans, staff development plans, administrative action plans, and all documentation. Process standards can and should be modified by health care professionals based on their judgment as the situation warrants.

This system of standards management which is inherent in THE BLUEPRINT, proves a great advantage in the event of litigation. The rules of THE BLUEPRINT are simple: structure standards (e.g., policies) are not situationally negotiable. When change is appropriate, structure standards must be renegotiated by the executive nurse council (see Chapter 4). Outcome, process, and evaluation standards are negotiable by the health care professional as the situation demands.

Evaluation

Evaluation standards are another innovative component of THE BLUEPRINT. They have always existed but typically have been unidentified. Just as standards must be set for acceptable operation of a health care facility and for acceptable delivery of care, so standards also must exist to delineate acceptable appraisal practices. Evaluation standards within THE BLUEPRINT include all appraisal mechanisms, tools, and research. Chapter 14 deals specifically with this type of standard.

■ KEEPING IT ALL STRAIGHT

To remember the broad-based categories of standards and to understand the terminology, think of quality assurance as a game:

- Structure—the rules of the game
- Outcome—the score, winning or losing the game
- Process—playing the game
- Evaluation—play by play analysis of the game.

■ ADVANTAGES OF THE BLUEPRINT

There are six advantages to using THE BLUEPRINT:
1. *It organizes system values.* The three domains organize standards into standards of care, practice, and governance. THE BLUEPRINT offers a logical definition of these standards.
2. *It enables the division of nursing to appraise its entire system.* Rather than focusing on patient care delivery in isolation, THE BLUEPRINT utilizes evaluation standards to establish methodology for appraising the entire division of nursing.

3. *It enables continual improvement of the division of nursing.* THE BLUEPRINT enables the organization to pinpoint the source of a quality problem or opportunity whether it relates to care delivery, the nursing staff, or the system in which care is taking place, or a combination of these. The model's action planning system tracks results of attempts to improve care, practice, and service. It provides a methodology by which problems can be isolated and improvements made in each domain.

4. *It enables the division of nursing to control its service.* Through its well-defined standards program, things happen the way managers want them to happen. That is control.

5. *It enables the division of nursing to control its costs.* By conservative estimate, 40% of the operating costs of a service business are spent on nonconformance. Tools and formats in this model are used to improve performance and thereby control costs.

6. *Accreditation requirements are fulfilled.* THE BLUEPRINT has been designed with an eye on the Joint Commission's agenda for change. It is in compliance with the current accreditation requirements and is in sync with the projected changes. It promotes a standard-based, performance management system that focuses on continual improvement in nursing services.

REFERENCES

1. American Nurses' Association: Publication G-124, p 4, 1976.
2. Brett JL: Outcome indicators of quality care. In Dimensions of nursing administration, theory, research, education, practice, Boston, 1989, Blackwell Scientific Publications.
3. Coyne C and Killien M: A system for unit-based monitors of quality of nursing care, J Nurs Admin 17:26, 1987.
4. Katz J and Green E: THE BLUEPRINT for quality management. In Schroeder P: Nursing quality assurance, vol II, Approaches to nursing standards, Gaithersburg, 1991, Aspen Publishers, Inc.
5. O'Leary D: The Joint Commission's agenda for change—stimulating continual improvement in the quality of care. Presented at American Organization of Nurse Executives preconference, Baltimore, May 14, 1990.
6. Peters T: Thriving on chaos, New York, 1988, Knopf.
7. von Oech R: A whack on the side of the head, New York, 1990, Warner Books, Inc.

3

TRANSITION: QUALITY ASSURANCE TO QUALITY MANAGEMENT

Nobody likes change but a wet baby.
ROY BLITZER

■ ABANDONING OBSOLETE POSITIONS IN QUALITY ASSURANCE

It is a well-known fact that horses, confronted with a life-threatening stable fire, cannot be easily made to leave the comfort and familiarity of their environment. The very sights, smells, and sounds of fire, which others recognize as signals to abandon the stable, compel the terrified animals to cling to familiar surroundings. One could say that the Joint Commission has initiated the fire of change in the stables of health care and there are a lot of frightened health care professionals who refuse to leave the stalls. These professionals seek comfort in the accustomed rituals of quality assurance within the health care stable unaware that they, like the horses, can survive only if they abandon their familiar positions!

Abandoning positions never before questioned is frightening. It involves change and, as Roy Blitzer says, "Nobody likes change but a wet baby."

The old adage "change takes time" is true. Change that occurs over a period of time is much easier to absorb into our thinking and incorporate into our lives. Everyone needs time to adjust to change.

In the health care industry today, however, changes are occurring with such swiftness that there is little time to adjust. An unsettled feeling pervades the health care industry—just ask any health care professional. A new procedure is barely initiated, the ink is barely dry on the newly designed QA tool, when there is notification of a new regulation or change in Joint Commission terminology. It is little wonder that many QA professionals feel like horses caught in a burning barn!

Survival, however, will depend on how well we adapt to the new health care environment, how willing we are to abandon obsolete positions. Some changes that have occurred include abandoning emphasis on auditing charts. Data collected by observation and interview are usually more accurate than data retrieved from a patient's chart. The word "audit" has been replaced by "evaluation." The familiar term "auditing of problems" has been replaced by "evaluating standards." In fact, the term "quality assurance" is under fire and rarely used today. In actuality, quality cannot be assured, only managed or improved. In today's environment it is preferable to think and speak about "quality management" or "quality improvement" instead of quality assurance.[5]

With all of these rapid changes in approaches and terminology, it is difficult for the health care professional to keep abreast of them. To survive the pressures of the changing health care environment, however, there must be a willingness to embrace change and abandon some long-held QA opinions.

Among opinions that must be reevaluated are these: QA is punitive; QA reports negative events; QA monitors tasks; charts are a major source of QA data; monitoring should be random; QA and standards are unrelated; and rationales are necessary for carrying out procedures, policies, and standards.

Punitive Quality Assurance

A good example of punitive QA is the practice of using incident reports as a basis for employee evaluations. The purpose of incident reports is not to evaluate employees, but to provide a vehicle for reporting deviations from "normal processes." The data compiled from incident reports should then be used to provide a thorough, accurate, and complete report of the deviations. Compilation of these data should be used for prevention of future deviations and for continual improvement in care and service.

If employees view incident reporting as punitive, however, they will tend to avoid punishment by concealing documentation that they perceive to be incriminating. Punitive action on employees who file incident reports will reduce only the number of *reported* incidents! A good example is the discrepancy between the number of reported medication errors on a research survey versus the number reported on hospital incident reports.[2,3] In the transition to quality management, the incident report's negative image must be eliminated. This can be accomplished only by the astute nurse manager who is willing to convert incident reports into positive tools for change. One way to do this is to avoid placing incident reports in employee files, where they become part of the employee's permanent employment record.

Negative QA Reporting

In the past, quality assurance often consisted of an accounting of the negative aspects of care and service. Hospitals often used the term "QA-ing" a problem, indicating that QA was synonymous with blame assessment.

It is time to focus on what is being done *right* within the organization and to use monitoring to validate the care being given. Managers who find that their staff members are noncompliant and uncooperative with the QA program need to reexamine the focus of the program. Quality can be a positive force, even in a busy department. Remember the principle: "What gets rewarded, gets done!" Then reward, in every possible way, the excellent work of each employee. The reward can be as simple as a sign on the bulletin board of the nursing unit that reads, "My thanks this week to _____ for _____," signed by the nurse manager. Where the organizational focus is positive—that is, where monitoring validates excellence—there is little difficulty in regarding quality as a part of the daily work experience of all staff members.

Monitoring Nursing Tasks

Previously, monitoring focused mainly on nursing tasks. A checklist was typically used as the data collection tool. If the nurse cleaned, rubbed, stuck, patted, and inserted according to policy and procedure, quality was said to be present; this was confirmed by an evaluator who observed the nurse's actions and then checked them off on a list. How comforting were those checklists for quality assurance! One popular checklist asked: (1) Is the arm band on correctly? (2) Is the bedrail up? (3) Is the chart labelled correctly? (4) Is the hallway free of clutter? Indeed, for many years such checklists were accepted. The problem with them was that while they confirmed that isolated tasks were performed properly, they failed to address the true issue, which was total patient safety, the outcome of the tasks. When the siderail was up and the arm band was placed correctly, the patient might still fall out of bed or be given the wrong medication. When tasks were monitored, the evaluator *still* could not prove that patient safety was adequate, for safety was and is a much broader issue than can be measured in isolated tasks.

For example, one hospital, wishing to decrease the incidence of falls, has implemented a patient safety practice program called the "red dot program." It is multidisciplinary in that all staff members—housekeepers, maintenance personnel, physicians, and so on—are involved. When a patient is identified as being at "high risk for falls," either on admission or at a later time, a red dot is placed on the patient's arm band, bed headboard, chart, Kardex, and room door. Every employee is responsible for preventing a fall by that patient. If a housekeeper is mopping the floor of a "red dot" room and notices that the bedrail is lowered, it is his or her responsibility to summon a nurse immediately. If a patient with a red dot is being transported within the hospital, every employee is responsible for that patient's safety. All employees are educated on their part in the "red dot program," and receive a list of reportable observations.

The new QM dictates that a practice guideline for patient safety be implemented that encompasses an organized plan for total patient safety. In the past, patient safety has been a singular *nursing* function. Realistically no one nurse is capable of observing every patient every minute. Together, however, the total health care team is able to ensure patient safety. Monitoring should then be directed toward the outcome of the management of patient safety by the team. This is a much different approach than having the nursing staff check off tasks completed on a list of "dos and don'ts."

Chart Review as Major Data Source

Chart reviews are excellent tools if the focus of the study is documentation. If, however, the goal is to improve care or service, chart reviews are of little value. In the transition to QM, nurse managers must seek methods of data retrieval and feedback that permit continual improvement in (1) patient care, (2) staff members' ability to function effectively, and (3) the administration's capacity to provide necessary support. Data sources should include, but are not limited to:

- Patient, staff member, manager, ancillary staff interviews
- Patient, staff member, manager, ancillary staff questionnaires
- End-of-shift report
- Problem logs
- Incident reports
- Infection control reports
- Quality Management Council analyses
- Direct observation
- Simulations

Random Monitoring

Monitoring that focuses exclusively on collecting volume indicators and auditing problems at random must be abandoned in favor of a planned, organized, systematic monitoring and evaluation program. Monitoring should focus on those aspects of care and service that are high risk, high volume, problem prone, and high cost. These terms will be explained further in Chapter 6. Additionally, there should now be a concrete, written monitoring plan along with a 3- to 5-year monitoring calendar.

It is impossible to monitor all facets of every aspect of care. Careful planning must therefore be undertaken to determine what is monitored, how often, why, and by whom. While unusual occurrences will be the focus of immediate and intensive reviews, all other data collection and evaluations must be well orchestrated by a knowledgeable quality management team. This promotes a cost-effective, successful quality management program.

QA Unrelated to Standards

Important aspects of care and indicators cannot be written unrelated to the standards of the division of nursing. The important aspect of care is identified first, then an indicator is developed. The indicator is derived from the standards that define care delivery in that important aspect.

For example, if the important aspect of care to be evaluated is identified as alterations in skin integrity related to pressure ulcers, the practice guideline that described the care and management of pressure ulcers would be used as the standard against which to measure quality. While tasks are incorporated into the practice guideline, it is a process standard that encompasses far more than tasks. The practice guideline uses the nursing process to delineate the assessment: when, where, and how often; the planning; the interventions; the evaluation; and the necessary competencies to carry out the care of the patient with the specific condition. The practice guideline is a complete patient management tool that includes outcomes in each domain. The outcome of this practice guideline in the clinical domain might be, "The patient will maintain or reduce the size of the pressure ulcer during length of stay." If monitoring validated that the outcome was met, quality care could be said to have been present clinically. The indicator to monitor might read, "The number of patients whose pressure ulcers maintained or reduced in size." For a detailed discussion of indicators, see Chapter 7.

Rationale

Written rationales are redundant. Whether written into procedures or policies, or attached to standards, they should be eliminated. For example, consider the following procedure, with accompanying rationale:

Procedure for application of electrodes for continuous monitoring. Rationale: In order to maintain proper contact between patient's skin and the electrode, application must be performed correctly.

This statement is cluttered with redundant information. The likelihood of staff members reading a standard is inversely proportional to its length. An unnecessary textbook rationale adds length and clouds the clarity of the standard. All "purpose" and "rationale" statements should be eliminated. It is expected that staff members know *why* they are implementing a standard, otherwise *they would not have initiated it in the first place.*

■ WHY CHANGE?

Organizational survival will depend upon the willingness to go beyond the quality assurance approaches that worked in the past and to embrace the new quality management concepts designed for the future. Health care professionals should change their approaches to QA for many of the same reasons that health care organizations have adopted electronic thermometers: it is faster, more efficient, and easier to use; it creates greater patient safety; and it is cost effective. Just as each member of the health care team had to learn to use the new thermometers, so each will have to learn to use the new quality management methods. THE BLUEPRINT is a model that will bring an organization into this new era.

The new quality management focus of the 1990s is on organization-wide programs. THE BLUEPRINT is a useful model to design such a program. It has made the old nursing-focused QA obsolete. This exciting new approach to total organizational quality has assisted a number of organizations to redesign their quality management program. Implementing THE BLUEPRINT creates opportunities for health care professionals to use innovative methods to improve patient care delivery, to work together as a team, and to control the costs associated with the delivery of care. THE BLUEPRINT facilitates development of multidisciplinary standards. It contains the formats necessary to guide the organization in writing standards, which may then serve as the benchmark against which to evaluate clinical, professional, and administrative progress.[4]

Change, however, is rarely easy. There is a natural tendency to resist deviating from the current, familiar quality assurance methodology. The new quality management approach is untried and frighteningly unfamiliar. Whereas previous QA programs focused on identifying problems, the new approach focuses on improving the norm of performance by creating a standards-based monitoring and evaluation system. A model such as THE BLUEPRINT can help an organization make the transition to this new approach.

■ NURSING AS A SERVICE DELIVERY BUSINESS

The infusion of business concerns into the nursing role, with emphasis not only on performance but also on productivity and outcomes, has permanently altered nursing. Today a master's degree in business administration (MBA) is more helpful to the RN seeking an executive management position than is a PhD.

Many health care professionals, including nurses, are bewildered in the new environment, with its complexities of corporate control and cost containment. This emphasis on business seems to be at variance with nursing's professional ideals; yet, there is no doubt that nursing is a business. The three basic components of business are present in the nursing profession: someone who receives a service, someone who delivers a service, and someone who governs the service.

In other words, three distinct domains are present: clinical, professional, and administrative. Each domain corresponds to a business component. THE BLUEPRINT is based on these three domains and provides a model for quality management within the division of nursing.

THE BLUEPRINT emphasizes the business aspects of nursing. Each practice guideline can be used to identify the cost of care. Each coordinated plan of care incorporates the patient's estimated length of stay based on the admitting diagnostic-related group (DRG). Incorporating the business aspects of nursing into THE BLUEPRINT is innovative and timely.

Why is this business perspective a necessity today? Many hospitals closed in the 1980s and more are projected to close in the 1990s. Faced with rising labor, equipment, and insurance costs, many hospitals are in financial difficulty. In this environment, a business orientation can have a tremendous impact on health care costs. This philosophy is incorporated into the standards and domains of THE BLUEPRINT. It is no longer possible to solve today's problems with yesterday's tools! THE BLUEPRINT is an up-to-date tool for quality management.

■ IDENTIFYING SOME OBSOLETE POSITIONS

It was inevitable that a business perspective would eventually be adopted by the nursing profession. When the prospective payment system was legislated in 1981 and implemented in 1983, money became a paramount issue in health care.

The prospective payment plan originated at Yale University as a management and utilization review tool. The federal government, seeking a method for controlling soaring health care costs, adopted the Yale plan as a solution. Within 3 months it formulated legislation that changed the health care industry and the nursing profession.

The prospective payment system allocates a predetermined payment for patient care based on the patient's DRG regardless of the actual costs of the care provided. Hospitals have a strong financial incentive to reduce the length of stay and thereby reduce their costs. As a result, nursing—already hurt by a severe nursing shortage—is called on to give more care to more acutely ill patients.

Nursing outcomes that include rehabilitating patients in the activities of daily living and in spiritual and psychological health are no longer achievable during the shortened hospitalization. As one nurse said, "I now have 3 days to achieve all the things I used to do in 7!" The challenge to nursing was to provide excellent patient care within the hospital's budgetary constraints. The short, controlled length of stay for each patient means that nurses have minimal time in which to achieve all the essential outcomes.

Under the new system, cost, as determined by the government, is a new factor. Everything done within the division of nursing must be justified in terms of costs and results. Process standards must be cost-effective and produce desired outcomes. The concepts of ideal standards and quality assurance, long held sacred, have vanished. Frequently, nurse managers are unprepared to meet the new challenges.

The quality assurance programs of yesterday were not designed to measure the multidisciplinary, complex care of patients with problems involving acute conditions medically or surgically, aging, immunosuppression, violence, and drug abuse. What can be done? Truly, the industry's stable is on fire! To survive, the nursing profession must reevaluate its earlier operating systems, such as, definition of standards, documentation systems, and policy and procedure development and use.

Documentation

Narrative Charting. Narrative charting is qualitative and not quantitative. Handwriting varies, so that retrieving data for evaluation or confirmation of testimony during litigation is difficult. In contrast, flow sheets or checklist charting are quantitative and easily measurable at a glance. In this age of cost constraints, staff shortages, and increased litigation, the profession cannot afford to write paragraphs of documentation when flow sheets have proven more efficient and are legally just as sound!

Duplication of Documentation. An item should be charted in one place in a patient's record. The human error associated with multiple entries could create a legally unsound document. Furthermore, the variations in recorded results negate the benefits of chart reviews as a data collection technique. The likelihood of a documentation error is directly proportional to the number of times an item is transcribed. Consider the number of times a single laboratory value is mentioned in a patient's chart!

Individualized Care Planning. Individualized care plans remain a fundamental part of health care organizations even though they are no longer required by the Joint Commission. However, these individualized care plans need to be restructured to include quantitative, measurable indicators that facilitate measurement of the care being provided. Care planning should rarely be narrative; it should be crisp, precise, and reflective of total care in a format that permits shift-to-shift measurement of accountability. The professional can no longer spend inordinate amounts of time in writing. A plan of care remains important—but it must be an integral part of the documentation system in a format that focuses on accountability for patient care results.

Kardex. In past years, nurses used small, blue medicine tickets to match patients and medication. These were carried from room to room and inserted into a slot in the tray containing the medications which had been prepared in the medication room. With the advent of team nursing, a new system, called the Kardex, was developed. One nurse, the team leader, made all assignments, gave all medications, and did all charting for an entire group of patients. The Kardex served as the central source of information from which to operate during the shift. While team nursing was discarded by most hospitals, the Kardex was not! Indeed, in many hospitals, four to six nurses can be seen during each shift, all clustered around the medication cart with the Kardex at the top. Each nurse is trying to use the Kardex and dispense medications—creating an in-house traffic jam.

The Kardex system is cumbersome and not user friendly, and gives rise to administrative and documentation errors.

To enhance the quality of the system, the Kardex should be replaced with individual medication records kept on clipboards at the bedside along with the patient's progress records, care plans, and admission records.

The recommended system is indeed for the convenience of the nurses!

Policy Development

Policies for Everything. Policies constitute the structure upon which monitoring is based. Policies are nonnegotiable directives that outline the dispensing of care, practice, and governance. A clear delineation of policy is mandatory.

Every "rule" or "wish" is not and must not be referred to as a policy. If a "rule" can be modified based on circumstances, it cannot be a policy. For example, changing dressings on a surgical wound is part of a practice guideline because it can be modified. However, identification of the personnel permitted to change dressings *is* policy because it cannot be modified. The inappropriate designation of "negotiable" rules as policies encumbers the quality management program and renders it less effective.

When negotiable and nonnegotiable rules are mixed, staff members may confuse the two and modify a nonnegotiable rule while following to the letter a "rule" that *should* have been modified. For example, a policy to restart IVs every 72 hours may result in an IV being discontinued in an 87-year-old patient with poor veins. Clearly, guidelines for restarting an IV are negotiable and should not be policy; the information belongs in a practice guideline. Policy, on the other hand, is *never* negotiable. For example, a patient in ventricular fibrillation may be defibrillated *only* by certified personnel.

Procedures. Procedures involve psychomotor skills. In general, clinical psychomotor skills are performed by staff members to or for patients. Each procedure is associated with a documented practice guideline that contains details of patient care and management. Valid procedures are a sequence of precise steps that can be used as indicators in the monitoring and evaluation process. Ideally, written procedures may be placed on 4- × 6-inch laminated cards. They should be as short and succinct as a cooking recipe. The only reason that some hospitals offer for creating lengthy procedures (one hospital displayed a 3-page procedure for passing ice water and a 6-page procedure for giving a bed bath in their 5-inch thick Policy and Procedure Manual) is to "satisfy Joint Commission requirements." Volumes of unmeasurable, repetitious, unusable requirements were *never* a mandate of *any* accrediting body. Procedure manuals should be designed for use by the staff, and should provide a quick reference.

Policy and Procedure Manuals. In their typical unwieldy form, policy and procedure manuals are rarely used by staff members, and often contain outdated information. Moreover, their typical form does not facilitate evaluation of either policies or procedures!

Massive policy and procedure manuals should be separated into two distinct documents. Policies are structure standards and procedures are process standards. Each must be developed and maintained independently for ease of staff reference, monitoring, and evaluation. Policy statements do not belong in procedures manuals and procedures do not require a policy for implementation.

■ UNDERSTANDING THE OUTCOME FOCUS OF QUALITY MANAGEMENT

Reevaluating and revamping familiar systems such as policy and procedure manuals can be unsettling as can be the new emphasis on *outcomes*. Many nurse managers ask how the outcome emphasis differs from what has been done in the past.

Outcome-focused quality management emphasizes quality in the broadest sense. It represents a fundamental change in the way evaluations and reviews are to be conducted. Continual improvement in care, practice, and governance is the underlying principle. Inherent in this strategy is the conviction that there must be consistent improvement in *everything* that is done and in the *way* it is done.

There is a new mandate: everyone in the organization takes part in quality management by setting standards to eliminate unnecessary work, simplify necessary work, and determine the results to be achieved. This necessitates the development of outcome-focused standards.

To write standards that are truly results oriented, the outcomes to be achieved must be incorporated into the written process standard. For every practice guideline and procedure (process standards), there is an associated outcome. For example, the outcome for the "Procedure for Assisting with the Insertion of a Chest Tube" might read, "The nurse will prepare the Pleurovac and suction apparatus and, using sterile technique, set up the chest tube procedure tray within 15 minutes of the physician's order for insertion." In all clinical procedures, the outcome should identify that which the *nurse* expects to achieve by implementing the standard.

If the standard is multidisciplinary, then the physician, nurse, respiratory therapist, and so on, should each have an outcome written on the standard specific to their specialty. The outcome may then serve as the basis for development of an indicator to monitor the standard. In this way, outcome-focused quality management addresses the degree to which an outcome is achieved by following the standard, as opposed to the traditional QA method, which focuses on tasks to be performed.

While the focus has shifted from monitoring the activity to monitoring the results, the results will demonstrate the appropriateness of the activities. When results, or outcomes, are monitored, the activities required within the standard become apparent. This permits continual improvement and refinement of standards, as well as a check on outcomes.

In other words, outcome standards cannot be divorced from process standards. To illustrate the truth of this statement, consider this story from Roger von Oech's book, *A Whack on the Side of the Head*. Several centuries ago, a curious but deadly plague appeared in a small village in Lithuania. What was curious about this disease was its effect on its victims; as soon as a person contracted it, he or she would go into a deep, almost deathlike, coma. Most died within a day, but occasionally a hardy soul would return to the full bloom of health. The problem was that since eighteenth-century medical technology was not very advanced, the unafflicted had a difficult time determining whether a victim was dead or alive.

One day it was discovered that someone had been buried alive. This alarmed the townspeople, so they called a town meeting to decide what should be done to prevent such a situation from happening again. After much discussion, most people agreed on the following standard: They would place food and water in each casket, next to the body. They would fashion an air hole going from the casket up to the earth's surface. Maintaining this standard would be expensive, but more than worthwhile if it would save lives. The outcome they hoped to achieve was: "The patient will be able to remain alive, even though buried, until someone is alerted and rescues him."

Another group came up with a second, less expensive standard. They proposed implanting a 12-inch stake in each coffin lid directly above the place where the victim's heart would be. Then, whatever doubts there were about whether the person was dead or alive would be eliminated as soon as the coffin lid was closed. The outcome of the second group's standard was: "The patient will be dead, when buried, forever."[6]

This story illustrates how standards are developed to achieve a specific outcome. It also illustrates that standards and outcomes may be inappropriate. Achieving the outcome is not always synonymous with quality.

■ INTEGRATING THE BLUEPRINT WITH THE TEN-STEP PROCESS

Two outstanding mechanisms are available to ease the transition from quality assurance to quality management: (1) the Joint Commission's ten-step process for Monitoring and Evaluation, designed to assist health care facilities to develop an effective QM plan, and (2) THE BLUEPRINT FOR QUALITY MANAGEMENT, designed to facilitate the implementation of the ten-step process. *Each will prove indispensable in the transition phase.*

Long-term success and survival in the increasingly competitive health care environment depend on quality management being implemented in the most cost-effective manner. The correct program must be implemented the *first* time. THE BLUEPRINT has been designed to ensure that the Joint Commission's ten-step process is implemented correctly the first time. THE BLUEPRINT contains all the necessary tools for using the ten-step process as the basis for developing a quality management program.

The Joint Commission's quality assessment standards emphasize the importance of planned, systematic, and ongoing monitoring and evaluation activities, and THE BLUEPRINT provides a framework within which those activities can occur. The transition phase will be simplified with use of THE BLUEPRINT.

The following is an overview indicating how THE BLUEPRINT simplifies the ten steps required by the Joint Commission in the monitoring and evaluation process.

Step 1: **Assigning Responsibility.** Each department director should be responsible for and actively participate in monitoring and evaluation. The director assigns responsibility for the specific duties related to monitoring and evaluation.

THE BLUEPRINT includes a unique controlled, shared governance council structure that clearly delineates all responsibility within the division of nursing. It separates nursing service into clinical, professional, and administrative domains, which lend themselves to council structure and a decentralized approach to quality management. The quality management council has authority for quality control within the division of nursing. This invests authority in the nursing staff, giving them accountability for their practice.

Step 2: **Delineating Scope of Care and Service.** Each department should establish an inventory of its clinical, professional, and administrative activities. This delineated scope of care/service provides a basis for identifying those aspects of care and service that will be the focus of monitoring and evaluation.

THE BLUEPRINT offers three tools to facilitate accomplishing this step. It also offers an outline for creating important patient, staff, and management profiles.

Step 3: **Defining Important Aspects of Care and Service.** Important aspects of care/service are those that involve high risk, high volume, high-cost activities, and/or problems. Staff members should identify important aspects in order to focus monitoring and evaluation of those areas having the greatest impact on quality of care.

THE BLUEPRINT includes grids, which serve as tools for quickly identifying high-risk, high-volume, problem-prone, and high-cost aspects of care and service. In addition, guidelines are provided for what and how much to monitor as well as how often.

Step 4: **Identifying Indicators.** Indicators of quality should be identified for each important aspect of care/service. An indicator is a well-defined, measurable ratio related to the structure, process, or outcome of care. Indicators should be objective and measurable and should help direct attention to potential problems or opportunities to improve care.

Within THE BLUEPRINT, a form for indicator development has been devised. Further, THE BLUEPRINT defines how these indicators should be monitored and evaluated by staff. They can be used to validate nursing's contribution to the organization's total quality improvement.

Step 5: **Establishing Thresholds for Evaluation.** Thresholds for evaluation are the levels or points at which intensive evaluation of care is initiated. A threshold should be established for each indicator. Thresholds should be based on statistical analysis.

In THE BLUEPRINT threshold parameters are set on the indicator development form for each individual indicator. The indicator development form is a hallmark of THE BLUEPRINT.

Step 6: **Collecting and Organizing Data.** Appropriate staff members should collect data pertaining to the indicators. Data should be organized to facilitate comparison with the thresholds for evaluation.

THE BLUEPRINT specifies that the departmental quality management committee identify the important aspects of care to be monitored and design the monitoring calendar and studies. Staff members collect and analyze the data. This written analysis is sent back to the quality management council for review.

Step 7: **Evaluating Variations.** Appropriate staff members should evaluate the care provided to determine whether a problem exists. This evaluation should be sensitive to possible trends and patterns of performance. The evaluation should also attempt to identify causes of any problems or methods by which care or performance may be improved.

A threshold parameter form is used to identify if individual study results fall within the desired limits and to determine if the important aspect of care is in statistical control over time.

Step 8: **Taking Action.** When problems are identified, action plans should be developed and approved at the appropriate levels and enacted to solve the problem or take the opportunity to improve care.

Action planning is an integral part of THE BLUEPRINT. Action plans are concrete tools that are part of the model. There is an action-planning tool for each domain:

1. To solve a clinical problem at the bedside, a clinical action plan is used.
2. To solve a professional problem with a member of the staff (e.g., lack of knowledge or motivation), the employee development plan is used.
3. To solve a problem in the system, the administrative action plan is used.
4. To solve a problem involving lack of knowledge about new technological equipment or new information, the staff development plan is used.

Step 9: **Assessing the Actions and Documenting Improvement.** The effectiveness of the actions should be assessed and documented. If further action is necessary to solve a problem, it should be taken and its effectiveness assessed.

A progress record tool for assessing actions and documenting improvement is an integral part of THE BLUEPRINT.

Step 10: **Communicating Relevant Information to the Organization-Wide Quality Assurance Program.** Findings from and conclusions of monitoring and evaluation, including actions taken to solve problems and improve care, should be documented and reported through established channels of communication.

Several methodologies have been developed within the framework of THE BLUEPRINT for communicating relevant data, including the quality assurance bulletin board and the end-of-shift report.

When THE BLUEPRINT is used to implement the Joint Commission's ten-step process, the transition from traditional quality assurance to contemporary quality management will be a smooth one. The chapters in Part Two focus on the use of THE BLUEPRINT in each step of the process.

REFERENCES

1. American Nurses' Association: Standards for organized nursing services and responsibilities of nurse administrators across all settings, Kansas City, Mo, 1988, ANA.
2. Francis G: Nurses' medication "errors": a new perspective, Supervisor Nurse 11(8):11.
3. Ludwig-Beymer P et al: The effect of testing on the reported incidence of medication errors in a medical center, J Continuing Educ Nurs 21(1):11.
4. Katz J and Green E: THE BLUEPRINT for quality management. In Schroeder P: Encyclopedia of nursing care quality, vol 2, Approaches to nursing standards, Gaithersburg, Md, 1991, Aspen Publishers, Inc.
5. O'Leary D: The Joint Commission's Agenda for Change—stimulating continual improvement in the quality of care, presented at AONE preconference, Baltimore, May 14, 1990.
6. von Oech R: A whack on the side of the head, New York, 1990, Warner Books, Inc.

Part Two

IMPLEMENTING THE TEN-STEP PROCESS

4

STEP 1:
ASSIGNING RESPONSIBILITY
FOR QUALITY

The buck stops here.
HARRY S TRUMAN

When Harry Truman was President of the United States, he kept a sign in the oval office that read "The buck stops here." If quality is to become a reality in today's complex health care organizations, there *must* be a place where the buck stops, and accountability for quality is acknowledged. Quality accountability has often been like the proverbial pea under the shell—now you see it, now you don't—an elusive component in health care organizations. Within many organizations quality is a delegated task. It is not an organization-wide commitment.

Quality management will be successful only if accountability starts at the top. W. Edwards Deming, the man credited with revitalizing Japanese industry, knew this. Mary Walton, in *The Deming Management Method*, recounts Deming's relationship with the Ford Motor Company:

In June 1980, when NBC aired its White Paper that featured Dr. Deming, *"If Japan Can . . . Why Can't We?"* the Ford Motor Company was in serious trouble. . . . It was clear that the nation's second-largest corporation had to change to survive. . . . The year Dr. Deming came to the attention of American industry was the year Ford lost $1.6 billion.

A copy of the NBC White Paper ended up in Ford's library of corporate self-help films. . . . William E. Scollard, then general manager of the automotive assembly division [watched the tape].

After seeing the tape, Scollard phoned the Ford quality department. 'Who is this Dr. Deming?' he wanted to know. He asked them to get in touch with the quality expert.

Dr. Deming, suddenly the object of much attention in corporate America, did not abandon his prerequisites merely because Ford was calling. He would work only where there was a commitment from top management, and he refused to come to Detroit unless his presence was requested by the president of the company.[2]

If today's health care organizations are to be quality minded, forging quality control into the driving force behind continual improvement, there must be a commitment throughout the hierarchy of the organization. This will mean rethinking and restructuring some organizations.

Imagine trying to renovate and update a pre–Civil War mansion: the first step would be to shore up the foundation and install modern wiring. Similarly, health care organizations must restructure their management foundations, and the division of nursing should function as the *prime* contractor in the renovation process. The division's foundation should be reinforced with *controlled shared governance* so that the "wiring" of council structure can take place. This council structure would then enable quality management, like electricity and heat, to permeate the entire structure.

In other words, a total systems reevaluation and, perhaps, overhaul is a prerequisite to assigning quality management responsibility. Each organization must design a management structure that makes the pursuit of quality a part of the daily work experience of all staff members, not just of management. This means, then, that the management style *must* be one that facilitates shared responsibility and accountability.

In the past, nursing management had accountability for quality assurance while nursing staff members had responsibility. Today, if quality management is to be used to reduce costs and improve care, it can no longer be limited to management's spot checking the work of the bedside nurse. While that may have been sufficient when hospitals were small and relatively simple organizations, it is no longer a practical approach.

Management must give nurses the authority to create standards to control care, mandate professionalism, and manage systems issues that affect care. Thus, responsibility and accountability for care, practice, and governance are invested directly in nursing staff members. If quality management is to become a realistic, organization-wide administrative tool for continual improvement of care and services, then it needs to have not only a division-wide thrust, but also specific staff member involvement.

The division-wide thrust to make quality a part of the daily work experience can be achieved by adopting a system of *controlled* shared governance in which *quality management* plays an obvious, continuous, and integral role through council structure. This council structure provides specific, realistic staff member ownership, participation, and accountability. When nurses "own" their clinical and professional practice their commitment to the organization is increased.

■ CONTROLLED SHARED GOVERNANCE

In today's litigious, cost-contained environment, it is mandatory that nurses accept responsibility and accountability for care, practice, and governance within the division of nursing. Indeed, the Joint Commission views this as step 1 of the assessment process. One of the best ways to meet the Joint Commission's requirement is to adopt the management style of controlled shared governance.

Controlled shared governance is a logical way to restructure an organization to ensure shared responsibility and accountability throughout all departments. It is called *controlled* shared governance because, though responsibility and accountability are invested in the staff members through council structure, the council is designed and appointed by management. In other words, the most qualified employees are chosen by management to fill the council chair positions. Unlike some shared governance models, no positions are obtained by popular staff vote.

Controlled shared governance is readily accepted by the staff because they are able to control both clinical and professional practice. The council structure is also accepted by the management because there are built-in checks and balances that preclude attempted "staff takeovers":

1. The executive nurse council (ENC) functions as a court of appeals when council conflicts arise.

2. The ENC appoints council chairs so that the most qualified and supportive personnel function in power positions.
3. Educators and clinical specialists serve on all councils lending clinical and professional expertise.
4. Interacting councils communicate relevant data.

Controlled shared governance can eliminate the fearful, adversarial relationship between management and staff that has developed in some shared governance systems. In the past, shared governance systems, which were designed to allow an RN to sit on the board by popular staff vote, were often perceived by hospital boards as attempted hostile nursing takeovers.

In controlled shared governance there is no attempt by staff members to wrest control of the organization from management, nor is there an attempt by management to sabotage staff members' assumption of their responsibility and accountability, because there are no turf battles to be fought. Council functions are well delineated, preventing organizational upheaval. Controlled shared governance works because not only is all responsibility and accountability for care, practice, and governance shared but it is also clearly delineated in writing.

In one organization that implemented controlled shared governance as advocated in THE BLUEPRINT, the Professional Practice Council functioned independently of management to solve a pressing problem. In this situation, staff members began arriving for work dressed in street clothing instead of professional uniforms. Management received numerous patient complaints of inability to distinguish care givers from visitors and/or other levels of workers. A need for a dress code was obvious.

Prior to controlled shared governance, management would have issued an ultimatum to staff: conform to our management-mandated dress code or seek employment elsewhere. Under controlled shared governance, the problem was referred to the Professional Practice Council for resolution.

Given this responsibility, the Professional Practice Council deliberated through several sessions and sought input from each nursing department. The council then established a reasonable dress code. All staff members understood that infractions of the code would be handled by this peer group in council session. Since no staff member wanted to appear before the council after having broken the code, the problem was solved.

■ ASSIGNING RESPONSIBILITY FOR QUALITY MANAGEMENT

Assigning responsibility for quality management is a daunting task in the absence of a guide or model. The controlled shared governance model provides a guide for restructuring responsibility and accountability through council structure. Making quality a part of the everyday work experience of all staff members becomes a reality under the management style of controlled shared governance.

■ ORGANIZATION-WIDE RESPONSIBILITY FOR QUALITY MANAGEMENT

While the focus of this book is quality management within the nursing division, it is important at this point to address the interaction between the division of nursing

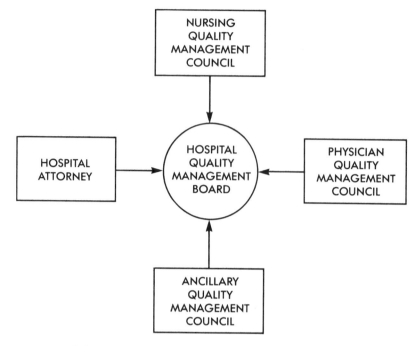

■ **FIGURE 4-1**   **Hospital quality management structure.**

and organization-wide quality management. It is a mistake to assign responsibility for quality management to nurses alone! Nurses do not make up an autonomous segment of the health care organization. In fact, all parts of an organization are connected; the quality of care or service in one part affects and is affected by the quality of care or service in all other parts. Quality management will be effective only when the separate components of the organization are directed toward the common purpose of quality improvement. Controlled shared governance, using organization-wide council structure, is a means to achieve that outcome.

Figure 4-1 illustrates how control of an organization's quality management can be invested in an organization-wide quality management board (QMB). The chair of this board is appointed by and reports directly to the chief executive officer (CEO) and sits on the hospital board of directors. The hospital attorney is also a member. The figure shows how nursing quality management fits into organization-wide quality management. Note that the QMB, which meets biannually, is composed of three councils—the nursing quality management council, the physician quality management council, and the ancillary quality management council—plus the hospital attorney.

The principal duties of this council include reviewing all high-risk incidents that occurred during the past year, improving standards to prevent recurrences of those incidents, and designing appropriate action plans to solve identified problems.

The chair and assistant chair of the three quality management councils meet quarterly for the following purposes: to communicate relevant data and disseminate organization-wide monitoring information; to provide a forum for interdepartmental, multidisciplinary, quality problem-solving; to prevent overlap in data collection or to provide an opportunity for creating multidisciplinary monitoring and evaluation; and to review all organization-wide clinical practice deviations (e.g., a Swan-Ganz catheter left in place longer than 72 hours, an endotracheal tube left in place longer than 5 days, and the like).

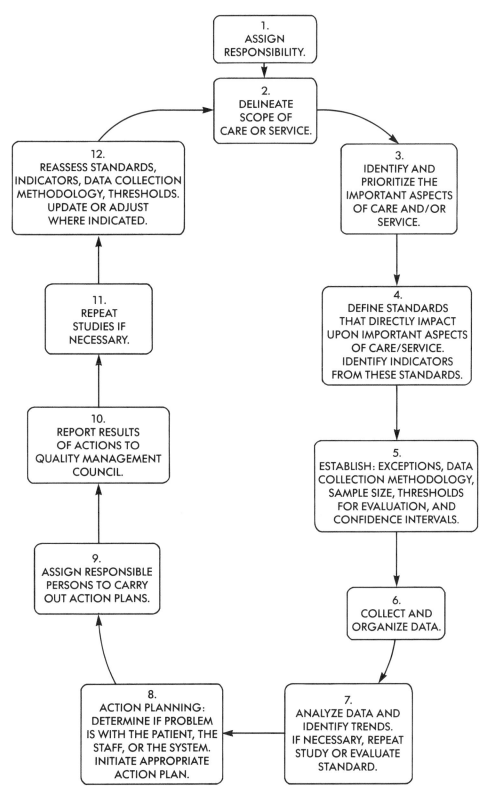

■ FIGURE 4-2 The quality improvement cycle.

This council structure provides an ongoing cycle of quality improvement throughout the organization, which is depicted in Figure 4-2. Note that steps 11 and 12 have been added to the Joint Commission's recommended ten steps.

■ ASSIGNING RESPONSIBILITY FOR NURSING DIVISION QUALITY MANAGEMENT

Controlled shared governance within the division of nursing permits nurses to maintain control and accountability for direct patient care, for professional practice, and for issues of governance that involve nursing. Furthermore, through council structure, nursing is able to monitor and evaluate patient care, professional practice, and nursing governance without usurping management and systems operation functions.

In today's health care organizations, the vice president for nursing is charged with the responsibility of facilitating, delineating, and establishing written standards of care, practice, and governance and for monitoring and evaluating those standards to continually improve care and service within the division of nursing. Nursing Standard NC.3.1.1 states that "the nurse executive has the authority and responsibility for establishing standards of nursing practice."[1] This can most easily be accomplished through council structure.

Also, there has been a change from the term "committee" to "council." A committee, according to *Webster's Dictionary,* is "a body of persons delegated to consider, investigate, take action, or report on some matter."[3] Thus, by definition, a committee cannot perform the duties necessary to manage and ensure division-wide quality.

The definition of council reflects today's quality environment. A council is "an executive body whose members are equal in power and authority."[3]

Nurse Council Structure

Figure 4-3 portrays the five councils that are necessary to organize and manage the division of nursing: the executive nurse council (ENC); the professional practice council (PPC); the administrative practice council (APC); the clinical practice council (CPC); and the quality management council (QMC).

The model in Figure 4-3 depicts four councils circling the QMC and feeding into a circle of conductivity. This circle is like the steering wheel of an automobile—driving, directing, and steering the division of nursing via its four council arms. The wheel enables reciprocal interaction among all councils as well as with the hub or center council, the QMC. The QMC is placed in the center of the wheel as the "horn" or alarm device, ready to sound at the first hint of trouble.

The council structure is effective because it provides the opportunity for each council to interact freely with all other councils. The QMC functions independently to coordinate the assessment, monitoring, and evaluation of the processes and outcomes of each domain—clinical, professional, and administrative—of the division of nursing.

Council Structure for Assigning Nursing Responsibility

Executive Nurse Council (ENC). The ENC is composed of the chairs of the other four councils. The ENC chair is the vice president for nursing who also sits on the

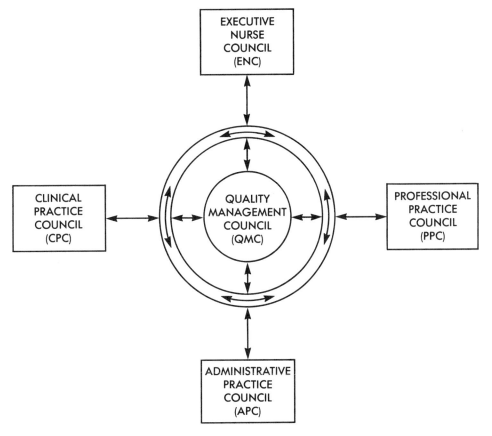

■ **FIGURE 4-3**   **Nurse council structure denoting the circle of conductivity.**

hospital board of directors and hospital executive committee. Figure 4-4 depicts the composition of the ENC, which meets monthly. Its duties include:

- Carrying out the corporate mission (e.g., developing division-wide philosophy and goals)
- Strategic planning of division of nursing (e.g., establishing priorities)
- Policy development (e.g., physical resource utilization and management)
- Determining the delivery of care methodology (e.g., acuity system, staff mix, use of agency personnel, sitters, private duty)
- Budget management/allocation of funds in the division
- Handling legal issues
- Contracting (e.g., student placement, consulting)
- Giving final approval to all nursing policies
- Marketing (e.g., public relations, community interface)
- Appointing council members

The ENC functions as the arm at the top of the wheel, which steers the division of nursing. The ENC plays a major role in controlled shared governance. It is the place where "the buck stops," where managerial and council effectiveness is evaluated and adjusted, and where alternatives and costs are considered in selecting courses of action for the division of nursing.

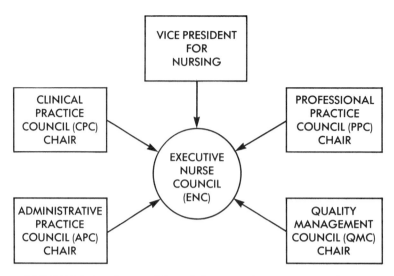

■ FIGURE 4-4   Composition of the executive nurse council (ENC).

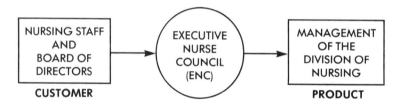

■ FIGURE 4-5   Customer and product of the executive nurse council.

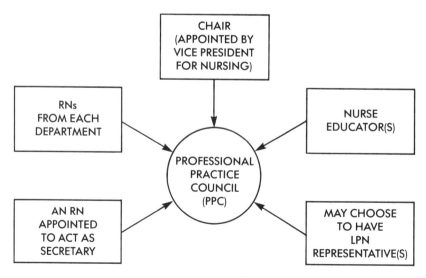

■ FIGURE 4-6   Composition of the professional practice council (PPC).

Each council assumes accountability to a customer and produces a product. The ENC maintains accountability not only to the division of nursing but also to the board of directors for the practice of nursing within the organization. Figure 4-5 illustrates the customer and product of the ENC.

Additionally, the ENC coordinates the work of all the other councils and acts as the arbiter for problem resolution when councils cannot resolve issues.

Professional Practice Council (PPC). The PPC is composed of one nurse from each unit of the division of nursing, depending on the size of the nursing staff. Additionally, two members of the education staff sit on this council. The council chair is appointed by the vice president for nursing. The council members are appointed by the ENC. Figure 4-6 depicts the composition of the PPC.

This council meets monthly. Its duties include:

- Supporting the corporate mission
- Supporting the division of nursing's professional practice philosophy and goals
- Establishing and writing professional practice procedures
- Establishing competencies on clinical practice guidelines
- Establishing and writing professional practice guidelines
- Overseeing continuing education (e.g., identifying staff educational needs)
- Overseeing professional recognition
- Managing the clinical ladder
- Establishing a dress code
- Resolving competency issues (e.g., professional credentialing or certification)
- Resolving conflicts among staff members
- Resolving collaborative practice issues
- Differentiating professional from technical practice
- Addressing professional ethics issues
- Participating in research
- Recommending action planning when necessary
- Resolving all problems dealing with professional practice within the division of nursing
- Overseeing peer reviews
- Overseeing professional documentation

The PPC functions as the professional arm that steers and directs all issues surrounding the professional practice of nursing. The PPC plays a major role in the controlled shared governance management structure because this council delineates the written standards for professionalism within the division of nursing. This council permits professional staff members to govern themselves, and to determine issues of competency, dress, behavior, and collaborative practice. Figure 4-7 depicts the customer and product of the PPC.

Administrative Practice Council (APC). The APC is composed of all head nurses, nurse managers—including first-line managers, shift coordinators, supervisors, resource nurses—and their assistants. A management position grants council membership. The council chair is appointed by the ENC and meetings are held monthly. Figure 4-8 depicts the council structure. Its duties include:

- Supporting the corporate mission
- Supporting the division of nursing administrative practice, philosophy and goals
- Writing administrative policies

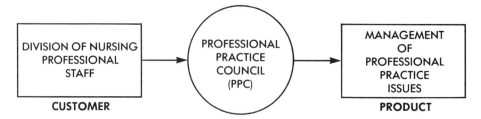

■ **FIGURE 4-7**   Customer and product of the professional practice council.

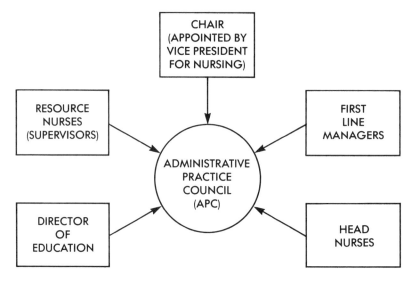

■ **FIGURE 4-8**   Composition of the administrative practice council (APC).

- Establishing and writing administrative practice procedures
- Establishing and writing administrative practice guidelines
- Overseeing the fire and safety committee
- Participating in research
- Recommending action planning when necessary
- Overseeing administrative documentation
- Writing job descriptions
- Managing equipment and supplies (e.g., linen, new products, repairs)
- Resolving operational difficulties
- Writing, distributing, and analyzing nurse manager satisfaction questionnaires
- Resolving day-to-day operational conflicts and problems

The APC is responsible for administrative practices, such as administrative policies, procedures, and practice guidelines within the division of nursing. In addition to the wide range of duties and responsibilities listed above, this council provides the managers with a forum for interaction. Figure 4-9 depicts the customer and product of APC.

Clinical Practice Council (CPC). The CPC is composed of one nurse from each unit in the division of nursing depending (as with the PPC) on staffing. Clinical specialists from the department of education are also members of this council. The council chair

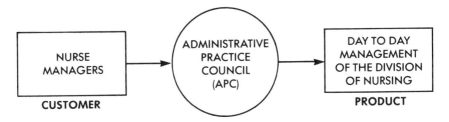

■ **FIGURE 4-9**   Customer and product of the administrative practice council.

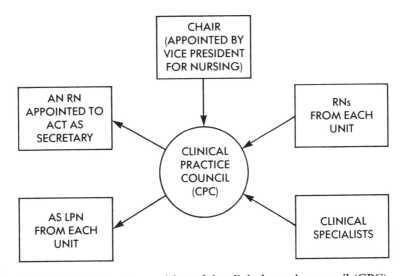

■ **FIGURE 4-10**   Composition of the clinical practice council (CPC).

and members are appointed by the vice president for nursing. Figure 4-10 depicts the composition of this council.

CPC meetings are held once each month. Its duties include:

- Supporting the corporate mission
- Supporting the division of nursing clinical practice philosophy and goals
- Approving the clinical standards for the division of nursing
- Coordinating the writing of all clinical procedures
- Coordinating the writing of all clinical practice guidelines
- Overseeing development of patient teaching plans
- Determining care planning methodology
- Determining all clinical documentation
- Developing action planning when necessary
- Interacting with infection control
- Participating in research

The CPC maintains accountability for all clinical practice within the organization. This council is invested with the responsibility of coordinating the writing of clinical practice standards and approving them. Figure 4-11 depicts the customer and product of CPC.

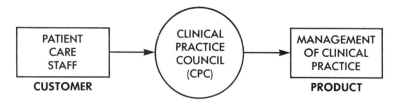

■ FIGURE 4-11   Customer and product of the clinical practice council.

Quality Management Council (QMC). In the controlled shared governance model the QMC is the hub around which all the other councils revolve. The quality management council replaces the old quality assurance committee.

The QMC is composed of a quality management coordinator from each unit of the division of nursing as well as two members from the education department. The coordinators play a vital role in the division quality management program because they oversee each nursing department's quality management program as assigned by the council. Once the data are collected, the quality management coordinators analyze the results and report the results to QMC. This permits systematic and routine comparative analysis of all monitoring and evaluation data within the division of nursing. Collaborative data analysis among all nursing departments is the by-product of this council.

The quality management coordinators will also chair task forces on their respective units to delineate scope of care and identify and prioritize important aspects of care. In addition, they will be responsible for coordinating and writing the department-based quality assessment plan according to the Joint Commission's Ten-Step Process. Certainly, the QMC is central to all quality management activity. Figure 4-12 depicts the composition of this council.

The QMC chair is appointed by the vice president for nursing. The council meets monthly. Its duties include:

- Writing and implementing the division of nursing quality assessment plan
- Identifying division-wide important aspects of care
- Delineating scope of care and service
- Establishing and maintaining division of nursing monitoring and evaluation calendar
- Coordinating all division of nursing monitoring and evaluation activities (e.g., setting up monitoring tools, determining sample size, setting thresholds, determining data collection methodologies, tabulating data, analyzing data)
- Recommending appropriate action planning
- Interfacing with hospital-wide quality management
- Conducting intensive reviews

QMC functions as the division of nursing's quality management hub. In addition to the monthly meetings, this council meets biannually with the hospital quality management board. The customer and product of QMC are depicted in Figure 4-13.

Processes, outcomes, responsibility, and accountability are not separate spheres, but interactive, dynamic elements. Each one is central to the quality of health care. When operating together, at every level, there is cohesion, fluidity, and precision. These principles should guide and gird the entire health care organization.

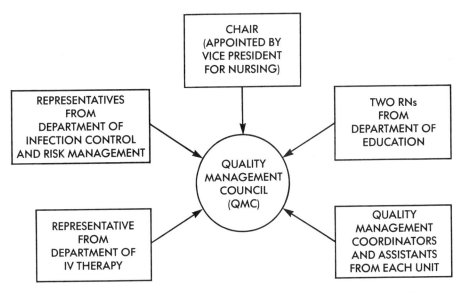

■ **FIGURE 4-12**   Composition of the quality management council (QMC).

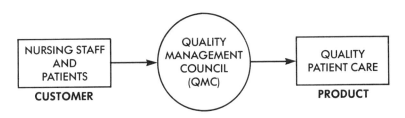

■ **FIGURE 4-13**   Customer and product of the quality management council.

Step 1 of the Joint Commission's ten-step process requires that an organization assign responsibility for quality management. This task is not difficult when the system is organized to facilitate quality management with efficient services, full utilization, and representation of all staff members, with planning and accountability central to the realization of the division of nursing's goals.

As never before, the health care industry is in the business of providing cost-effective, health-effective patient care. The challenge is for the industry to reorganize its various parts into a functioning whole in order to achieve maximum quality, organization-wide accountability, and fiscal responsibility. That challenge can be met when management is by controlled shared governance.

REFERENCES

1. New nursing care scoring guidelines, Joint Commission Perspect 10(4):B1-B46, 1990.
2. Walton M: The Deming management method, New York, 1986, Putnam Publishing Group.
3. Webster's Ninth New Collegiate Dictionary, Springfield, 1983, Merriam-Webster Inc.

5

STEP 2: DELINEATING SCOPE OF CARE AND SERVICE

If you don't know where you are going,
when you get there, you don't even know you're there.
HERB COHEN

Perhaps you've read the poem about the six blind wise men who wanted to learn about elephants, so they visited one. But, because they were all blind, they could not see the elephant. Each wise man touched a different part of the elephant to determine what the animal felt like; each man drew a different conclusion:

- The first stumbled into the elephant's side and decided that an elephant is like a wall.
- The second touched the elephant's tusk. He compared the elephant to a spear.
- The third held the elephant's trunk and concluded that elephants are similar to snakes.
- The fourth felt the elephant's leg and decided that elephants are very much like trees.
- The fifth felt the elephant's ear and determined that elephants resemble fans.
- The sixth, who grasped the elephant's tail, claimed that all elephants are like ropes.

The poem concludes:

And so these men of Indostan,
Disputed loud and long,
Each in his own opinion
Exceeding stiff and strong.
Though each was partly in the right,
And all were in the wrong!*

A similar behavior is sometimes manifested by those seeking to delineate the scope of care and service (step 2 of the Joint Commission's ten-step process) in health

---

*John Godfrey Saxe's well-known fable appears in many collections, including *100 More Story Poems*, selected by Elinor Parker, New York, 1960, Thomas Y. Crowell Company.

care organizations. Because the organization is so large and complex and each manager is most familiar with the inner workings of his or her own department, there is a tendency toward fragmentation in delineating scope of care and service. The whole is seen only from a biased perspective.

When fragmentation occurs, important aspects of care and service may be overlooked in the monitoring and evaluation process and, even worse, an opportunity to improve is missed.

Step 2 is critical in the Joint Commission's ten-step process. Unless this step is thoroughly completed, step 3, which involves prioritizing the most important aspects of care and service, cannot be completed.

To complete step 2, the step should be divided into two distinct parts: the customer, and care and service. (See Figure 5-1.) If either component is missed, this critical step will be incomplete and will affect the organization's ability to implement the remaining eight steps of the ten-step process.

■ KNOW THE CUSTOMER

If true quality improvement is to occur, then quality *efforts* require a new way of thinking about the *customer*. Why focus on the customer? Because, as quoted in Zemke's *The Service Edge*, John Guerra, an AT&T branch manager, states, "Quality is not measured by me. It's not even measured by you. Quality is in the eyes of your customer."[4]

Who is the customer of a health care organization? The typical answer, "the patient," is only partly true. Health care organizations that believe that the patient is their *only* customer are mistaken.

Many customers exist within the organization. Before delineating the scope of care and service, the customers must be identified. It is important to know to whom the care and service is directed. When the customer is identified, it becomes easy to delineate the care or service each customer receives.

Identifying Each Customer

Using the three domains helps identify the customer. The customer in the clinical domain is the patient, the patient's family members, and the community. The customer in the professional domain is the staff, physicians, and ancillary staff. The customer in the administrative domain consists of managers, vendors, and administration. (See Figure 5-2.)

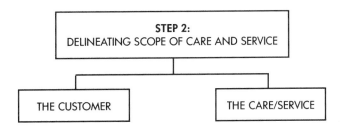

■ **FIGURE 5-1   For step 2 to be meaningful, it must be divided into two distinct areas: the customer, and care and service.**

CLINICAL DOMAIN (STAFF)	PROFESSIONAL DOMAIN (MANAGERS)	ADMINISTRATIVE DOMAIN (ADMINISTRATORS)
PATIENTS FAMILIES COMMUNITY	STAFF MEMBERS PHYSICIANS ANCILLARY STAFF	MANAGERS VENDORS ADMINISTRATION

■ FIGURE 5-2   Identification of customer domain.

Viewing the patient as the *only* customer indicates that the organization has addressed only the clinical domain. The customers in the professional and administrative domains have been ignored. A complete, total quality management program must have a tri-focus.

In the early 1980s many hospitals, following the lead of Memorial Hospital of South Bend, Indiana, assumed that the patient was everyone's customer and insisted upon "guest relations" training for all employees.[4] It soon became clear, however, that simply renaming patients "guests," in the Disney tradition, and conducting "Smile, staff, smile!" courses had little effect on the organization. Why? Because only the customer in the clinical domain was being addressed in the program; no mention was made of the professional and administrative domains. It is a grave business error in today's environment to believe that the health care organization's only customer is the patient.

From a business perspective, it is imperative to delineate clearly who the customers are in all three domains: clinical, professional, and administrative. How can an organization improve customer service if the customer is unknown? Companies such as Disney, Frito-Lay, and IBM have identified the importance of internal customers and used this knowledge to their advantage in becoming service leaders.[3] Remember, "quality is in the eyes of your customer."

But what does delineating the customer have to do with quality? Consider this fundamental rule: *with the customer as the reference point, priorities for action in each domain are easy.*

In other words, irrespective of domain, all quality management activities revolve around the customer. This means that all employees of the organization have an understanding of their customers in order to identify the scope of service. Furthermore, the customer within each domain should be clearly identified in writing as shown in Figure 5-2. Health care organizations must recognize their customers in each domain because this delineation allows for targeted program development, identifies areas of difficulty, and facilitates problem solving when customer complaints arise.

Traditionally, customer complaints in any domain other than clinical have been ignored because they were not viewed as *customer* complaints but, rather, as unavoidable staff disgruntlement, more to be accepted and tolerated than given serious consideration. Often staff complaints were not given serious consideration because health care organizations had abundant resources of time, money, personnel, and patients at their disposal. This abundance gave rise to the cavalier attitude that nurses were "a dime a dozen" and that there would always be sickness, trauma, and death, and a surplus of physicians and ancillary staff members. Few observers could have predicted the national economic chaos and nursing shortage that challenge the health industry today. After decades of this "take it or leave it" approach, many health care organizations find that their survival today depends on adopting different tactics.

In a recent study, Russell C. Coile, Jr., and Randolph M. Grossman asked the *Healthcare Forum* "panel of 300" to anticipate what is new and what is next "in the coming 1,000 days" for American health care. Overwhelmingly, the panel's answers revolved around quality—both quality of care and quality of caring. As described in *The Service Edge* by Zemke, Coile and Grossman concluded that measurement and the ability to "prove" customer satisfaction will be increasingly important.[4] However, before customer satisfaction can be "proven," there must be a clear understanding of who the customer is, and that means identifying every customer in each of the three domains.

In order for health care organizations to delineate their scope of care and service, the customer must be known in each domain. In quality-minded organizations, the meaning of the term "customer" must be broadened to include all who are users of the organization.

In every health care organization, there are external and internal customers. In the clinical domain, the patient, the patient's family, and the community are the external customers. However, there are internal customers in the professional and administrative domains too. If they go unrecognized, the organization's financial status and productivity will suffer. When an organization pays no attention to staff satisfaction, employees leave. This will result in the increased costs, diminished productivity, and lack of organization and loss of continuity of care and service associated with high staff turnover rates. An "every man for himself" mentality instead of a team effort where people care about the other "players" will devastate organizational morale.

THE BLUEPRINT assists in identifying all customers of a health care organization: the internal and external customers in the clinical domain, in the professional domain, and in the administrative domain. While the concept of the patient as a customer has long been accepted, the notion of identifying *both* internal and external customers is new.

Internal customers are just as necessary for the perpetuation of the business as external customers. Today, the combination of too few beds, too few dollars, too few nurses, and fewer patients—who have ever increasing expectations and demands—is shaking health care organizations to the core.[4] In this environment, *all* customers of the organization become vitally important. Recognizing customers in all three domains is critical to a quality transformation within the health care organization.

The Customer in the Clinical Domain. Typically, a department defines its scope of service by listing all the types of patients that are admitted. While this provides a general overview of the patient populations seen, it does not provide specific information about high-volume patients. These are the patients who make up the top three DRGs or medical diagnoses admitted to the department. They consume the most resources and thus additional information about these groups is needed.

Before delineating scope of care and service in the health care organization, there must be an understanding about who receives most of the care or service in that department. Knowing the intended recipient in the clinical domain controls or dictates how the care or service will be delivered. For example, a patient profile that reveals that the most frequently admitted patients have a diagnosis of chronic obstructive pulmonary disease, are male and homeless, and are primarily alcoholics with less than a third-grade education will influence how care and teaching must be carried out in this setting. There must be a plan of care that is tailored to this patient population. For example, handing one of these patients a pamphlet on chronic obstructive pulmonary disease and returning 30 minutes later for a "discussion" would be inappropriate. In this setting, specific, simple teaching plans should be developed using numerous illustrations and few, simple words.

Furthermore, understanding the customer in the clinical domain enables the organization to channel resources appropriately. For example, if a majority of patients cared for by the organization are poorly educated and do not speak English, resources expended to create a sophisticated patient satisfaction questionnaire written in English would be wasted—even if it were an award-winning project—because it would be inappropriate for the organization's typical customer. Instead, such an organization should create a simple satisfaction questionnaire to be used by the staff during patient discharge to record patient responses about their care and the hospital's services. Likewise, designing a follow-up call system may be inappropriate if the patient population is largely indigent.

In addition, knowing the intended customer assists health care organizations to predict appropriate outcomes of care and establish thresholds for evaluation of their service. For example, if the emergency department sees a very high number of IV drug abusers, an IV therapy standard that specifies that the IV should be started with one stick would be inappropriate because in many types of patients it may be virtually impossible to insert a needle into a vein in one stick. Furthermore, a standard such as

---

AV. AGE: _____ SEX: _____ MARITAL STATUS: _____ EDUCATION: _____

PERSONAL HABITS IMPACTING ON RECOVERY: _____

_____

COMMON MEDICAL/NURSING TREATMENTS:

   Diagnostic: _____

_____

   Therapeutic: _____

_____

   Medications: _____

_____

SOCIOECONOMIC STATUS: _____

COMMON COMPLICATIONS: _____

_____

COEXISTING CONDITIONS: _____

_____

POSSIBLE EMERGENCIES: _____

_____

PRIORITY NURSING DIAGNOSES: _____

_____

_____

■ FIGURE 5-3 Patient profile.

"no infections resulting from IV therapy" could prove unachievable for who can determine the cause of infection in a vein of an addicted patient who has abused every accessible vein?

For these reasons delineating the scope of care and service should not be attempted until a preliminary customer identification has been accomplished and a patient profile completed. A patient profile should be completed in each nursing department for the top three diagnostic-related groups or medical diagnoses admitted to that unit. This will provide a useful picture of the majority of the patient populations in each nursing department at any given time. Figure 5-3 presents an example of a patient profile. Any meaningful accreditation process includes a review of the patient profiles in order to assess care, practice, and governance in relation to patient population.

The patient profiles for the top three DRGs or medical diagnoses of a particular department should be maintained in the department quality management manual under step 2 of the Joint Commission's ten-step process. They should be reviewed and/or updated annually.

The Customer in the Professional Domain. While most health care organizations have little trouble identifying the patient as the customer in the clinical domain, they often have trouble identifying customers in the professional and administrative domains. Furthermore, while many have programs that emphasize treating patients as valuable customers, some might question the need for treating nursing staff as valuable customers. As one vice president for nursing service stated, "It's never occurred to me that the staff are also customers. The idea of catering to a professional staff member as though they are a valuable customer is a brand new thought. I'll have to think it through."

Even though high turnover contributes to increased operational costs, the management of some health care organizations refuses to link the turnover rate to their methodology. Fortunately, not all hospitals fall into this category.

Beth Israel Hospital in Boston, Massachusetts, is prominent among the hospitals that are systematically changing the personal involvement and professional status of their nursing staffs and viewing them as valuable customers of the organization.

In *The Service Edge* Ron Zemke points out the soundness of their reasoning: "Day to day, hour by hour, it's the nursing staff that does the business of the hospital, from checking vital signs and delivering medications to giving baths and answering questions from patients and family. Good nursing care has a direct, if often subtle, impact on everything from the satisfaction level of doctors (who these days can choose to put their patients in any of a number of increasingly competitive hospitals) to the willingness of a former patient to whistle up a lawyer when something doesn't turn out right. The nurse's knowledge, training and frontline experience is too valuable a resource to ignore. Hospitals are adjusting, and many of them are following the lead of that hospital out in Boston."[4]

Survival of many health care organizations today may depend on recognizing the health care professional as a customer. Trend tracker John Naisbit has predicted that by the turn of the century, as many as 2,000 hospitals will have either closed their doors or been absorbed into other hospital systems.[4] Meanwhile, the health care system is experiencing a growing deficit of registered and licensed nurses that, by some predictions, will reach 20,000 to 50,000 in the same period.

What is to be done to retain staff members and maintain safe, effective, and appropriate nursing care? Surely, managers of health care organizations must begin to view their staff members as their customers and treat them accordingly. Furthermore, departments within an organization must be recognized as each other's customers. For example, the recovery room would be the customer of surgery.

Dr. Arthur Kaplan, Director of the Center for Medical Ethics at the University of

Minnesota states in *The Service Edge,* "We have expectations of health care providers that have never existed before. We have yet to come to grips with the difficult choices that go with these demands."[4] Before nurse managers can "come to grips with the difficult choices" spoken of by Dr. Kaplan, they must first know their customer—the staff member. This means that each department manager identifies his or her professional customer in a formal, organized manner. This is accomplished in THE BLUE-PRINT through use of a staff profile.

A staff profile is a composite tool to assist in recognizing the customer in the professional domain. This profile, which averages staff data, is used for the following:

- The values of the organization can be matched with those of the staff members.
- The values of the staff members can be matched with those of the patient clientele.
- The experience and qualifications of the staff members can be matched with their expected role or job description.
- Employee development opportunities can be planned in accordance with needs of the staff members.

The staff profile should be maintained in the department quality management manual under step 2 of the Joint Commission's ten-step process. It should be reevaluated and updated every 3 years. Figure 5-4 depicts a sample staff profile.

The Customer in the Administrative Domain. In today's health care organizations, the nurse manager is often overlooked as a customer. Yet managers are the most valuable customers and resources of the administration. To overlook this can result in a vicious circle of nonproductivity and corporate negativity that pervades the organization. Management morale affects the overall perception of the organization by the public it is designed to serve.

The concept of the nurse manager as the customer of the administration of the health care organization is critical to corporate success in today's competitive environment. Yet, there is little documented evidence that nurse managers are cultivated as

AV. AGE: _____ SEX: % Male _____ % Female _____

MARITAL STATUS: % Married _____ % Single _____ % Divorced _____

EDUCATIONAL LEVEL: % LPN _____ % 2-yr _____ % 3-yr _____ % BS _____

   % MS _____ % PhD _____

% PART-TIME _____ % FULL-TIME _____ % FLOAT POOL _____ % PER DIEM _____

YEARS OF EXPERIENCE _____ CLINICAL LADDER LEVEL _____

PERSONAL HABITS IMPACTING ON EMPLOYMENT: _____

_____

SOCIOECONOMIC STATUS: _____

NUMBER OF CHILDREN: _____

TRANSPORTATION TO AND FROM WORK: _____

LENGTH OF EMPLOYMENT AT THIS FACILITY: _____

■ **FIGURE 5-4   Staff profile.**

valued customers of the administration. Each nurse manager represents a sizable investment by an organization. As Betty Holcomb points out in *Nurses Fight Back,* the cost of hiring and orienting a professional nurse for an organization has been estimated at $20,000.[2] Connie Curran states that the cost of turnover in the U.S. hospital industry in 1988 was *$3.2 billion.*[1] These costs do not include the time that colleagues spend helping to orient the newcomer to the organization, and all the other resources expended in helping the newcomer gain proficiency. Over time, the total investment in a nurse manager, in terms of formal and informal training, is very great. Despite this, organizations often allow these vital participants in the health care industry to run down, become technically obsolete, or burn out because they fail to recognize them as valuable customers.

Health care organizations often expend much effort on personnel or human resources. Practically all of them have active recruitment and retention programs. However, they expend only limited efforts on the *maintenance* of nurse managers. It is a rare organization that polls its nurse managers on a regular basis to solicit their opinions and assess their job satisfaction or that amasses a manager profile that identifies the characteristics of the majority of its managers. Many organizations operate without a fundamental knowledge of a primary customer in one of their domains. Nurse manager groups can vary in experience, longevity, academic preparation, and style.

A nurse manager profile can assist the organization to identify this important customer. Figure 5-5 presents a sample nurse manager profile. Organizations that know their management team profile can match potential managers with organizational values, discern compatibility with staff members' values, and estimate the professional's potential productivity based on home environment and other commitments, as well as the person's interest in personal and professional growth.

A manager profile should be part of the divisional quality management program and should be maintained in the quality management manual under step 2 of the Joint Commission's ten-step process. Department managers can use an adaptation of this profile for their charge nurses.

AV. AGE: _____   SEX: % Male _____   % Female _____

MARITAL STATUS: % Married _____   % Single _____   % Divorced _____

EDUCATIONAL LEVEL: % LPN _____   % 2-yr _____   % 3-yr _____   % BS _____

   % MS _____   % PhD _____

% PART-TIME _____   % FULL-TIME _____   % FLOAT POOL _____   % PER DIEM _____

YEARS OF EXPERIENCE _____   CLINICAL LADDER LEVEL _____

PERSONAL HABITS IMPACTING ON EMPLOYMENT: _____

_____

SOCIOECONOMIC STATUS: _____

NUMBER OF CHILDREN: _____

TRANSPORTATION TO AND FROM WORK: _____

LENGTH OF EMPLOYMENT AT THIS FACILITY: _____

■ FIGURE 5-5   Nurse manager profile.

	PATIENT (CLINICAL DOMAIN)	STAFF (PROFESSIONAL DOMAIN)	SYSTEM (ADMINISTRATIVE DOMAIN)
ROUTINELY OFFERED	1. Medication administration 2. Skin care 3. Pain control 4. Patient safety 5. Transportation within facility 6. Documentation of care 7. Use of nursing process 8. Infection control	1. Orientation 2. Preceptorship 3. Clinical ladder 4. Cross training 5. Employee documentation records 6. Written standards for practice 7. Controlled shared governance 8. Product orientation 9. Employee evaluation 10. Certification	1. Staffing 2. Acuity system 3. Admission/Discharge Practice Guidelines 4. Documentation system 5. Budget management 6. Hiring, firing, recruitment, retention practices 7. QM Program 8. Licensed personnel 9. Controlled shared governance
REQUESTED/AS NEED ARISES	1. Patient teaching 2. Security	1. Clinical inservices 2. Educational reimbursement 3. Weight loss clinic 4. Baby sitting service 5. Performance counseling 6. Management development 7. Maternity leave	1. Float/Agency personnel 2. Intensive review sentinel events 3. Employee health screens
EMERGENCY	1. Resuscitation 2. Spiritual counseling	1. Stress counseling 2. Spiritual counseling 3. Ethics counseling	1. Emergency staffing 2. Opening/Closing beds 3. Disaster teams

■ FIGURE 5-6 Matrix tool to delineate the scope of care and service of the division of nursing.

	PATIENT (CLINICAL DOMAIN)	STAFF (PROFESSIONAL DOMAIN)	SYSTEM (ADMINISTRATIVE DOMAIN)
ROUTINELY OFFERED	1. Medication administration (all routes) 2. Skin care 3. EKG monitoring 4. Use of nursing process 5. Documentation 6. 1:2 ratio nursing care	1. Staff safety 2. Orientation 3. Preceptorship 4. Certifications: Basic EKG, ACLS, IABP, IV therapy 5. Written standards for CCU 6. Clinical ladder 7. Controlled shared governance 8. Employee evaluation	1. Committee work: standards development 2. Peer review 3. End-of-shift report 4. Q Program 5. Participation in controlled shared governance
REQUESTED/AS NEED ARISES	1. Ratio of 1:1 nursing care 2. Hemodynamic monitoring 3. Pain control 4. Ventilator care	1. Cross training 2. Employee counseling	1. Intensive review of sentinel events
EMERGENCY	1. Bolus therapy 2. Advanced cardiac life support	1. Sick leave 2. Maternity leave	1. Emergency staffing 2. Triage in-house patients with chest pain on 11-7 shift. 3. Run EKG in-house on 11–7 shift.

■ FIGURE 5-7   Matrix tool to delineate scope of care and service of a specific department (in this example, coronary care).

■ DELINEATING SCOPE OF CARE AND SERVICE

Once the customers are identified and profiles are completed, the process of delineating scope of care and service can begin. This step is extremely important because it functions as the cornerstone on which the other steps are built.

To help delineate the scope of care and service, THE BLUEPRINT offers a matrix tool. (See Figures 5-6 and 5-7.) This tool should be completed and placed in the department quality management manual under step 2.

The matrix tool to be used to delineate the scope of care and service is organized vertically into the three domains: patient, staff, and system. It is organized horizontally into three divisions: routinely offered, requested/as need arises, and emergency.

If the matrix tool is being used to delineate the scope of services division-wide as illustrated in Figure 5-6, then three questions must be asked:

1. What does the division of nursing offer the patient?
   a. Routinely
   b. As requested or as need arises
   c. In an emergency
2. What does the division of nursing offer the staff members?
   a. Routinely
   b. As requested or as need arises
   c. In an emergency
3. What does the division of nursing offer the administration?
   a. Routinely
   b. As requested or as need arises
   c. In an emergency

To delineate the scope of care and service in a specific nursing department, simply fill in the name of the nursing department at the top of the page and repeat the process as outlined above. Figure 5-7 presents the matrix tool completed for a coronary care department.

Using the patient profiles and the matrices provides an organized, systematic, and planned approach to step 2 of the Joint Commission's ten-step process. It is the logical precursor to step 3, which is to prioritize the care and service that have been delineated in step 2. The prioritized items of step 3 are referred to as the important aspects of care and service, and they will become the focus of monitoring and evaluation described in the remaining chapters.

REFERENCES

1. Curran C: Keynote address: critical care update, issues, trends, and opportunities, National Conference Resource Applications, Inc, October 18, 1990.
2. Holcomb B: Nurses fight back. In Lindeman CA and McAthie M, editors: Readings in nursing issues and trends, Springhouse, Pa, 1990, Springhouse Publishing Co.
3. Peters T and Waterman R: In search of excellence, New York, 1982, Harper & Row Publishers.
4. Zemke R: The service edge, New York, 1989, Penguin Books.

6

STEP 3:
DEFINING IMPORTANT ASPECTS
OF CARE AND SERVICE

Our systems invariably measure "the wrong stuff."
TOM PETERS

Imagine a fantastic smorgasbord. The tables are overflowing with scrumptious food, everything "from soup to nuts." You are famished, and the mere sight of all that good food starts your salivary glands working overtime. This food fantasy, however, could be a nightmare if you are not careful. Falling prey to one of the following food traps could result in a gastronomic disaster.

The first trap is going on a binge. With reckless abandon, you attack the tables overloading your plate. You eat until you can eat no more. The error here is over-indulgence, and the lack of self-control results in a tight waistband and the burning desire for an antacid. You forgot that "all you can eat" does not mean you have to "eat it all." What should have been a satisfying experience has deteriorated to an unpleasant feeling of discomfort.

This also occurs when you try to overload your monitoring plan. This monitoring style represents an "eat it all" mentality. The misconception is that you have to monitor everything you do multiple times every year. The result is a monitoring plan that is unmanageable. "More" is not necessarily "better."

Every time a problem arises, regardless of its importance, it is added to the monitoring plan. Staff becomes frustrated with the volume of monitoring to be done. In an attempt to streamline the process and appease staff, you reduce the number of monitoring activities. This binge-purge cycle creates an unstable monitoring program. Staff begins to question the value of monitoring activities when the activities are important one day, and are discontinued the next. Like overeating, overmonitoring can transform what should be a positive, validating activity into an unpleasant experience.

The second food trap is grazing. Everything looks great. You want it all but do not want to overeat so you taste "a little bit" of everything. Your plate overflows with bits and pieces of many different foods. Soon you are full, but you have not had your fill of any one food. You want to go back to the table for more of something that you enjoyed but your stomach is too full.

In quality management there are grazers, too. This school of thought suggests that you monitor a little bit of a lot of things in an attempt to obtain a full picture of your services. There are two key problems with this approach. First, you may sacrifice monitoring something essential to monitor an activity of lesser importance. Second, you scatter your quality management resources, with little gain. The misconception is that everything you do must be monitored every year. You want to be sure that no matter what is examined, it involves some monitoring and evaluation activity. Dividing the monitoring time over so many issues usually means that all issues are treated the same. However, some parts of your service require more frequent and intense monitoring.

Indecisiveness is the root of this quality management trap. The result is a monitoring program that does not provide enough information to identify problems and initiate change. This indecision often stems from not knowing who the major customer of the service is and what key aspects are critical to achieving the desired patient outcomes.

In the final food trap, you indulge your "sweet tooth." You skip the meal and head right for the dessert table, discovering the strawberry shortcake and cherries jubilee. You fill up on empty calories and sacrifice good nutrition for palate pleasure.

Similarly, monitoring superficial indicators is a common quality management trap. It usually results from a misunderstanding of which elements of your service are most critical to the outcomes you need to accomplish. It is an attempt to keep data collection easy. The activities monitored may have little impact on the quality of your service. Staff becomes frustrated with the monitoring, perceiving it as busy work instead of meaningful analysis.

Just as your body requires a nutritionally sound diet to ensure effective functioning, your department requires a sound monitoring plan to ensure its effectiveness. Eating a balanced diet is a means to good personal health, and implementing a well-balanced quality management program is a key to good organizational health. A balanced diet is based on the four basic food groups. Similarly, a well-balanced monitoring plan is based on four important aspects of your service. These include the high-risk, high-volume, problem-prone, and high-cost aspects of your service.

■ IMPORTANT ASPECTS OF SERVICE

Tom Peters advocates keeping measurement simple—determining what variables capture the strategic essence of the department.[3]

Important aspects are those activities that are central to your service. They are the clinical, professional, and administrative activities that add value to your service and for which your service is valued. For example, in a hospice department, pain management is vital to palliative care. The competence of the nurses practicing in any given department is also a critical variable in delivering quality patient care: ". . . the ability of a health care professional or other staff to perform or support a patient care activity in the correct manner (i.e., without fault or error) and to perform or support the correct patient care activity (i.e., conforms with or adheres to preestablished guidelines) often has a direct bearing on quality of patient care."[1]

System variables also play a major role in determining the quality of patient care. Inadequate staffing and incompetent management may affect the quality of patient care as much as a drug error or nosocomial infection would. "One of the prerequisites for improving an organization's clinical performance is organizational and management effectiveness."[1]

The important aspects in the clinical, professional, and administrative domains are all critical to successful outcomes and patient satisfaction. Ignoring any of them jeopardizes the quality of your service.

The important clinical aspects of care vary from nursing department to nursing department based on the patient population and services provided. For example, important aspects of care for a patient with a fractured hip would differ from those for a patient with asthma.

The important professional and administrative aspects of care also vary from department to department. Important issues for a critical care department will differ from those for a hospice. While high-tech credentialing and one-to-one staffing may be important in critical care, they may not be significant for hospice.

Important aspects of care are also situational. They may change as the patient's acuity changes. Important aspects of care vary from the critically ill stage to rehabilitation. In critical care, activities geared to life support and physiologic stabilization are paramount. In rehabilitation, activities that promote restoration of function and adaptation of life style take precedence.

Professional and administrative importance is situational, too. High turnover and inexperienced nurses may be an important aspect of service one year but not the next.

The Joint Commission defines an important aspect of care or service as: "the diagnostic, preventive, therapeutic, rehabilitative, supportive, and/or palliative patient care activities or services within the scope of care or service of an organization, division, or unit that are of greatest significance to the quality and/or appropriateness of patient care."[2] This broad definition encompasses all types of institutions providing health care services from acute care to extended care facilities.

The key phrase in the Joint Commission's definition is "of greatest significance." While nurses like to believe that everything they do for patients is important, only those activities that are appropriate to the patient's condition and essential to achieving the desired results are of greatest importance. Choosing only the important aspects of care to monitor streamlines the appraisal process and makes the best use of resources.

Some activities are important because we do them frequently. Others are important because they are associated with significant risk or expense. Some are fraught with difficulties and, therefore, are labelled "problem prone." The important aspects of care that should be monitored can be categorized as high volume, high risk, problem prone, and high cost.

Determining important aspects of care requires knowing the customer. To determine important clinical aspects, one must focus on the patient. Every successful business considers its customer when developing its product or service. The customer in health care is the patient with a particular medical problem. It is critical that nurses understand to whom they are providing care because the important aspects of that care are determined by the patient's medical problems. By identifying the most commonly seen DRGs or medical diagnoses, the nurses in a specific department, whether in-patient or ambulatory, can begin to define the important aspects of the nursing services provided. This helps ensure that the services identified are appropriate to the majority of patients seen. Chapter 5 discusses the process of identifying customers and delineating scope of care and service.

High-Volume Activities

High-volume activities are those that occur frequently or those involving a large number of patients, staff, or nursing departments. However, high volume does not always indicate an important aspect of care. We may give numerous bed baths, but their significance to the patient's recovery depends on the type of patient and his or her acuity. A bed bath may not be an important aspect of care for a patient with a myocardial infarction, but may be of greatest significance to a patient with a large draining wound.

If over 50% of any of your top three DRG groups receive a particular service, that service should be considered high volume. If 25% to 50% of those patients receive the service, it is of medium volume, and if less than 25% receive the service, it is of low volume. Likewise, if a service is delivered once per shift or more to patients in any of the top three DRG groups, it is high volume. More often than once a week but less often than once per shift is medium volume, and once a week or less often is low volume.

In a medical-surgical department, chest auscultation and arterial blood gas analysis may be identified as priority diagnostic nursing services for patients with chronic obstructive pulmonary disease (COPD). In this department, chest auscultation is performed at least once per shift on all patients with COPD as part of the nursing practice guideline for managing the patient with impaired gas exchange. Improvement in the patient's oxygenation is monitored using this technique. Because the service is provided frequently to a large number of patients in a high-volume DRG and because it is appropriate to their condition and essential to track improvement, it is a high-volume activity. On the other hand, arterial blood gas analysis is performed only if the patient's condition deteriorates. It is not performed routinely and is not performed on more than 50% of the COPD patients. Although it is critical to positive outcomes, it cannot be considered a high-volume activity. It may, however, be classified as another type of important aspect of care.

Department-based orientation is an example of a high-volume staff activity. Every employee must be oriented. A professional practice activity should be considered high volume if it affects over 50% of staff in any given position or if the activity occurs frequently. "Frequently" is defined as once a week or more. If an activity occurs less than once a week but at least once a month, it is of medium volume. Those activities occurring on a quarterly basis or less are low volume. Other examples of high-volume staff activities might include CPR training and documentation. Again, regardless of frequency, activities are considered "important" only if they directly affect results. Likewise, high-volume administrative activities include those aspects that affect a large number of staff or occur frequently. Scheduling and patient classification are high-frequency administrative activities.

High-Risk Activities

High-risk activities include those in which harm or lack of significant benefit may occur either if the activity is performed or if it is not performed, i.e., acts of commission and acts of omission. An activity is high risk if its performance or omission could result in trauma, death, litigation, or loss of accreditation or license.

Chest auscultation is not usually considered high risk as it is not invasive in nature and its omission does not directly result in adverse reactions. Drawing arterial blood gases, on the other hand, could be considered high risk as it is an invasive procedure with the potential for infectious and bleeding complications. Other examples of high-risk patient care activities might include administration of potentially lethal medications, invasive monitoring, and CPR. High-risk staff activities would include failure to ensure CPR certification or lack of needle precautions. Administrative activities that may be considered high risk include a quality management program, staffing, annual licensure validation, and product evaluation. In each domain of practice there are activities that can be categorized as high risk.

Problem-Prone Activities

Problem-prone aspects of service include those activities that produce problems for the patient, the staff, or the system and/or those patient or staff populations that are prone to experience problems. Examples of problem-prone activities might include administration of chemotherapy, use of restraints, and pressure ulcer care. Examples of problem-prone patient populations might include geriatrics, immunosuppressed patients, and chemically dependent patients. Chest auscultation is not generally considered to be problem prone nor is arterial blood gas analysis. However, either of these activities may be labeled problem prone if there have been significant problems associated with providing the service or if there have been adverse patient outcomes. Problem-prone staff activities might include credentialing, the dress code, professional conduct, and use of nursing diagnosis. Examples of problem-prone staff populations might include graduates from other countries and new graduates. Administrative problem-prone activities might include patient classification systems or budgets. Impaired nurses or unionized employees might be examples of problem-prone groups from an administrative perspective.

High-Cost Activities

Health care costs in the United States have risen to over 11% of the gross national product (GNP). Some estimates suggest that medical expenses could escalate to more than 15% of the U.S. GNP by the year 2000.

High-cost aspects of service are not always obvious. It is easy to identify the very expensive items such as the use of specialized beds for skin care; however, small costs, if amassed in high volume, can significantly deplete resources. High-cost aspects of patient care services might include preventive skin care, fall prevention, and sterile procedures. High-cost staff services may include orientation, CPR certification, and continuing education. In the administrative area, absenteeism, use of agency personnel, scrubs, and overtime use may be examples of high-cost aspects.

■ CATEGORIZING SERVICES

An activity may fall into one or more of the categories of important aspects of care. For example, if a service includes oncology patients, administration of chemotherapeutic agents may be high volume because of the number of patients receiving it, high risk because of the toxicity of the agents, and problem prone because of their numerous side effects. It may also be high cost because of the cost of the drugs themselves and the equipment used and the fact that the nurses administering them must be credentialed.

In reviewing your scope of services, categorize the major patient care activities into the four types of important aspects of care. The form presented in Figure 6-1, "Important aspects of patient care," can help you organize your thoughts. Remember, an activity can fall into any or all of the categories. The importance of the activity and the need to monitor its impact on patient care services is directly proportional to the number of categories into which the activity fits. The form presented in Figure 6-2 can be used to list the professional and administrative important aspects of care.

Once you have categorized all aspects of your patient, professional, and administrative care or services, it is time to set priorities for monitoring.

DEPT: _____	DRG:	DRG:	DRG:
HIGH RISK	1. 2. 3. 4. 5. 6. 7. 8. 9. 10.	1. 2. 3. 4. 5. 6. 7. 8. 9. 10.	1. 2. 3. 4. 5. 6. 7. 8. 9. 10.
HIGH VOLUME	1. 2. 3. 4. 5. 6. 7. 8. 9. 10.	1. 2. 3. 4. 5. 6. 7. 8. 9. 10.	1. 2. 3. 4. 5. 6. 7. 8. 9. 10.
PROBLEM PRONE	1. 2. 3. 4. 5. 6. 7. 8. 9. 10.	1. 2. 3. 4. 5. 6. 7. 8. 9. 10.	1. 2. 3. 4. 5. 6. 7. 8. 9. 10.
HIGH COST	1. 2. 3. 4. 5. 6. 7. 8. 9. 10.	1. 2. 3. 4. 5. 6. 7. 8. 9. 10.	1. 2. 3. 4. 5. 6. 7. 8. 9. 10.

■ FIGURE 6-1   Important aspects of patient care.
(© 1991 Jackie Katz and Ellie Green. Reprinted with permission.)

	PROFESSIONAL	ADMINISTRATIVE
HIGH RISK	1. 2. 3. 4. 5. 6. 7. 8. 9. 10.	1. 2. 3. 4. 5. 6. 7. 8. 9. 10.
HIGH VOLUME	1. 2. 3. 4. 5. 6. 7. 8. 9. 10.	1. 2. 3. 4. 5. 6. 7. 8. 9. 10.
PROBLEM PRONE	1. 2. 3. 4. 5. 6. 7. 8. 9. 10.	1. 2. 3. 4. 5. 6. 7. 8. 9. 10.
HIGH COST	1. 2. 3. 4. 5. 6. 7. 8. 9. 10.	1. 2. 3. 4. 5. 6. 7. 8. 9. 10.

■ **FIGURE 6-2   Important aspects of service.**
(© 1991 Jackie Katz and Ellie Green. Reprinted with permission.)

Sentinel Events

A sentinel event is a serious, undesirable, and often avoidable process or outcome of patient care.[1] Sentinel events are of such significance and seriousness to the patient, the family, the practitioner(s), and the health care organization that an intensive review of each case must occur. To illustrate the gravity of a sentinel event, consider the following story. The resource nurse went with the local mortician to the morgue of a city hospital to release a body. On lifting the body onto the mortician's stretcher, the patient moaned. A code was called and the patient was transferred to the intensive care unit (ICU) where he survived for the next 5 days. This clearly is a sentinel event. Whenever a code is called in the morgue, an intensive review of what happened is warranted. Other less dramatic, but certainly important, examples might be falls resulting in injuries that prolong hospitalization or self-extubation resulting in respiratory arrest. A sentinel event concerning medication administration might be extravasation of a chemotherapeutic agent. If the activity is patient-controlled analgesia, a sentinel event might be death related to respiratory depression. In the nursery, dropping a baby is a sentinel event. An example of a staff sentinel event might be drug or alcohol use, or theft. An administrative sentinel event might be a fire or a staffing crisis.

Traditionally, a sentinel event was called an incident. In the past, however, incidents typically were labeled randomly and retrospectively. The advantage to anticipating the sentinel events associated with the important aspect of your service is that steps can then be taken to minimize the chances of their occurrence.

A list should be made of events that are considered to be serious enough to warrant an intensive review each time they occur. This list should become part of your department monitoring plan.

Establishing Priorities

To establish priorities for monitoring, first mark your completed grids (Figures 6-1 and 6-2) to delineate sentinel events. Then review the grid and list all the patient care services/activities that fall into all four categories for each of your top three DRGs. Services/activities that appear in all four categories have the greatest impact on your service and receive the highest monitoring priority. They are *critical* aspects of care. These activities will form the basis of your monitoring plan. For the patient with colorectal cancer in the oncology department, chemotherapeutic administration might be a critical aspect of care. The use of the intraaortic balloon pump for the acute MI patient, or suicide precautions for a psychiatric patient might constitute critical aspects of care. The authors suggest that these aspects be monitored at least quarterly.

Activities that fall into three of the four categories are *extremely* important aspects of care. They are the next level of monitoring priority. Aspects that fall into three of the four categories should be prioritized as follows:

1. *High risk, problem prone, high volume.* Examples include medication administration to stroke patients in a geriatric department or long term facility, or ventilator care for the ICU patient who has had coronary artery bypass graft surgery.
2. *High risk, problem prone, high cost.* Examples include care of the patient who is ventilator dependent or on hemodialysis.
3. *High risk, high volume, high cost.* Examples include administration of parenteral nutritional therapy or hemodynamic monitoring.

4. *Problem prone, high volume, high cost.* Examples include dermal ulcer care and blood administration.

These aspects should be monitored at least three times per year.

Staff examples of extremely important aspects might include the impaired nurse, preceptorship, and licensure validation. Administrative activities might include patient classification, the use of agency personnel, turnover, and absenteeism.

Activities that fall into two of the four categories are *very* important aspects of care and require monitoring at least twice a year.

Review the grid and list those activities that fall into two of the four categories according to the following priority order:

1. High risk, problem prone
2. High volume, problem prone
3. High cost, problem prone
4. High risk, high volume
5. High risk, high cost
6. High volume, high cost

Finally, list the activities that fall into only one of the categories. These are important aspects of care that should be monitored at least yearly.

It will be virtually impossible to monitor and evaluate all of your services/activities every year. To do so would require two staff members for every activity, one to perform the task and the other to monitor. Remember, the purpose of the monitoring and evaluation process is to spot check those activities that are most critical in defining the quality of your service. The cost of administering your quality management program is, of course, an important concern. Therefore, it may take 5 years to monitor all of the activities that you provide as services.

Narrowing Options

Once your list of priorities is completed the next step is to decide which of the activities will be monitored for each year of your 5 year plan. Choose one fourth to one third of your activities as those to be monitored. Of the topics chosen for monitoring 60% should be clinical, 20% should be professional, and 20% should be administrative. These will be the activities from which indicators will be chosen. (These monitoring guidelines are discussed in greater detail in Chapter 8.)

Each year you will review both the scope of services and the important aspects of services grids to validate and/or amend them based on any changes that have occurred in your services, staff, or patient populations.

By completing this step, you have laid the foundation for your quality management plan. The first three steps are the most time consuming, but once completed they serve to streamline the rest of the process. Well-defined responsibilities, well-differentiated scope of services, and important aspects of care are the key to developing a quality management program that monitors the essence of your services. They eliminate the haphazard, "knee-jerk" activities that can occur when monitoring becomes a response to isolated instances or specific situations. You will be assured that your monitoring plan is on target with the priority activities of your department and that those priority activities are consistent with your purpose.

REFERENCES

1. Joint Commission on Accreditation of Healthcare Organizations: Characteristics of clinical indicators, Quality Rev Bull, pp 330-339, November 1989.
2. Patterson C: Standards of patient care: The Joint Commission focus on nursing quality assurance, Nurs Clin North Am 233:625-637, 1988.
3. Peters T and Waterman R: In search of excellence, New York, 1982, Harper & Row Publishers.

7

STEP 4:
IDENTIFYING INDICATORS

Toto, I don't think we're in Kansas anymore!
THE WIZARD OF OZ

In the classic film "The Wizard of Oz," when the farmhouse finally lands and Dorothy steps through the door, you know immediately that something has happened. Up to that point, the film was shot in black and white. As Dorothy opens the door and steps through, the beautiful technicolor world of Munchkinland appears. The director used color as an indicator of a significant change.

Indicators are ubiquitous. They are positive or negative signs of change. Indicators measure various things. On a piece of machinery, an indicator monitors its function. The gas gauge in your car measures how much fuel is in the tank, thereby indicating approximately how many miles you can travel until you must refuel. In meteorology, indicators monitor the weather. A rise or fall in barometric pressure indicates a change in the weather pattern. In chemistry, indicators such as litmus paper measure the presence of a substance such as an acid or a base.

Indicators alert you—they forecast a deviation from the norm and may warn of impending problems. Economists pay special attention to indicators such as interest rates, unemployment rates, and inflation as predictors of an impending recession. Signs of a labor shortage are evidenced by higher vacancy rates, increased help wanted ads, increased retention activities, and higher salaries.

Indicators are a part of daily life. The clock indicates whether we are early, late, or on time. The calendar indicates the month, date, and day of the week. Traffic signals indicate stop, go, or caution, and a growling stomach indicates that it is time for a meal.

Just like "Hail to the Chief" heralds the arrival of the president and the first robin is the harbinger of spring, indicators may represent something else. They may not be a direct representation of measurement. While "Hail to the Chief" is not the president and the first robin is not spring, when you hear the first notes of that song or see the first robin, you know the president or spring has arrived.

We use indicators in health care, too. There are many clinical indicators. Some are direct measures; others are not. Vital signs generally indicate overall patient status. A thermometer directly measures body temperature, while the presence of a fever, rapid pulse, and increased respirations may signal an infection. Cyanosis, nasal flaring, and retractions suggest inadequate oxygenation, while arterial blood gas analysis confirms it by direct measurement.

■ INDICATORS IN QUALITY MANAGEMENT

In quality management "indicator" refers to a particular type of measurement. According to the Joint Commission, an indicator is a performance measure.[5] Performance is composed of competence and productivity. Competence means that the individual or organization has the ability to provide quality services. Productivity means that those abilities are translated into appropriate actions that achieve quality results.

Traditionally, the Joint Commission surveyed the capabilities of an organization—its competence. Was the organization able to provide quality care? Today, however, the thrust of the Joint Commission's accreditation activities has shifted to productivity, or the yielding of favorable results. No longer do the Joint Commission's surveys focus on the question "Is the organization able to provide quality services?" but rather, "Does the organization provide quality services?" For example, rather than deciding solely whether an institution follows a program to prevent patient falls, the reviewer will evaluate whether that program has any effect on the number of falls associated with injuries.

Indicators are critical tools for focusing on the desired outcomes and the essential processes for achieving quality outcomes. To date, the Joint Commission has focused on indicators related specifically to patients. They define a clinical indicator as "a quantitative measure that can be used as a guide to monitor and evaluate the quality of important patient care and support services."[2] It is not a direct measure of quality but rather a flag that points to specific issues that require more intensive review. Indicators enable organizations to monitor patient outcomes as a function of individual and organizational performance.

According to the Joint Commission,[2] an indicator is an event. It is expressed as the number of events compared to a specified universe of events. The ratio is expressed as:

$$\frac{\text{Number of patients for whom a specified event occurs}}{\text{Number of patients with the condition or procedure}}$$
the indicator is measuring

For example:

$$\frac{\text{Number of patients with acquired stage IV pressure ulcers}}{\text{Number of patients with pressure ulcers}}$$

or

$$\frac{\text{Number of urinary tract infections in patients with indwelling urinary catheters}}{\text{Number of patients with indwelling urinary catheters}}$$

Formerly, the Joint Commission used "indicator" to define the topic of the study and "criteria" to describe the specific questions that were asked about that topic. In the new terminology of the Joint Commission, "indicator" denotes the specific process activities and/or outcomes critical to an important aspect of care. For example, formerly the indicator might have been pressure ulcer care, and the criteria might have included the incidence of acquired stage IV ulcers. Now, however, the indicator is the number of patients with acquired stage IV pressure ulcers. Criteria have been replaced with *data elements*. The composition of the data elements varies with the type of indicator being monitored. Data elements are covered in Chapter 8.

Categories of Indicators

An indicator is categorized by the type and seriousness of the event it measures. The type of event measured by an indicator may be structure, outcome, or process and is clinical, professional, or administrative in scope. It may also relate to either the quality or the appropriateness of an event. *Seriousness* relates to the gravity of the event.

Types of Events

Structure, process, or outcome. Events may be structure, process, or outcome. Structure refers to the rules that govern how the service is provided. Process encompasses all of the activities provided and outcomes are the results of the process. For example, structure defines all the equipment necessary and available to perform surgery, process is how the surgery was performed, and the outcome is the success or failure of the surgery. For the process of patient education, structure relates to the necessary teaching aids; process is the act of patient teaching, and outcome is whether the patient learned.

Structure indicators are derived from the written structure standards. These standards include the mission, philosophy, goals, and policies of the division of nursing. Structure indicators measure whether or not the rules of the division are being adhered to. For example, if the important aspect of care being monitored is safety and the clinical policies states that all patients who are in a wheel chair or on a stretcher must have a seat belt on, a structure indicator might read,

$$\frac{\text{The number of geriatric patients up in a wheel chair with seat belt on}}{\text{Total number of patients up in wheel chairs}}$$

Process indicators measure specific aspects of the nursing process that are critical to patient outcomes. Examples of process indicators include assessments, routine and emergency treatments, and management of complications.[2]

Process indicators are derived from written process standards. These include the procedures, practice guidelines, plans, and documentation that outline how care is to be delivered and recorded. Process indicators may be used in conjunction with outcome indicators or in situations in which an outcome is not readily achievable in a time frame relevant to the organization. Pain management in terminally ill cancer patients is an example of a process indicator. Eradicating the cause of the pain to alleviate it is not feasible; therefore, pain control becomes the best available indicator of the process of managing the pain. It may be written:

$$\frac{\text{The number of patients with terminal cancer experiencing}}{\text{The number of patients with terminal cancer}}$$
$$\frac{\text{pain who achieve a satisfactory level of pain control}}{\text{experiencing pain}}$$

Outcome indicators measure what does or does not happen to the patient after something is or is not done.[2] These results may be desirable or undesirable. Outcome indicators are based on the written outcome standards that have been integrated into the process standards for the management of patient care. For example, the outcome for the venipuncture procedure might be to establish venous access in one stick. The outcome indicator would read:

$$\frac{\text{The number of one-stick venipunctures}}{\text{The number of venipunctures ordered}}$$

On a safety practice guideline, the outcome might be to avoid level IV falls, i.e., unsupported falls resulting in injuries. In this case, the outcome indicator would read:

$$\frac{\text{The number of level IV falls in geriatric patients}}{\text{within 4 hours of sedative administration}}$$
$$\frac{}{\text{The total number of level IV falls}}$$

Clinical, professional, or administrative indicators. The type of event measured by an indicator may also be categorized as clinical, professional, or administrative. A clinical event relates to an aspect of patient care. It measures key factors in the care that a patient receives or the outcomes of that care. For example, there is no evidence of physical injury to the patient as a result of application and maintenance of physical restraints. A professional event relates to an aspect of professional practice affecting patient outcomes. It measures key factors of professional practice that have an impact on the quality of patient results. For example, there is evidence of the use of the nursing process in each nurse's practice. An administrative event deals with organizational factors that affect patient outcomes. It measures key aspects of the system that affect the results of care delivery. Examples of administrative events include understaffing, bed utilization, and availability of equipment.

Clinical, professional, and administrative indicators can measure structure, process, or outcomes. Examples of clinical structure, process, and outcome indicators have been stated above. The number of nurses attending CPR classes is a professional process indicator. The number of nurses correctly initiating CPR in a code situation is a professional outcome indicator. An example of an administrative structure indicator is the number of times staffing was planned using the acuity system.

Clinical indicators are based on clinical standards; likewise, professional and administrative indicators are based on their respective standards. These indicators are just as important as the clinical indicators in determining quality of care. If not enough nurses are present in the department on a given shift, the clinical standards will not be met regardless of how well they are written. Similarly, if there are a sufficient number of nurses, but an insufficient number of them possess the requisite knowledge or skills, the clinical standards are meaningless.

Quality and appropriateness. Indicators also measure the quality and appropriateness of the service provided and the results obtained. Quality indicators deal with the effectiveness, timeliness, efficacy, efficiency, continuity, and consistency of care. The above examples are quality indicators. Appropriateness indicators measure whether the activity that is prescribed and/or performed is truly warranted by the patient condition. The quality may be good while the appropriateness may be poor. For example, a patient once placed in a therapeutic bed tends to be kept there even though this may no longer be indicated. Other examples of appropriateness indicators might be the number of times defibrillation was performed because of life-threatening ventricular arrhythmia, the number of times staffing was not appropriate to meet the identified needs of the patients, or the number of times in-service classes relate to specific needs identified through monitoring and evaluation activities. Both quality and appropriateness indicators should be a part of monitoring and evaluation activities. Inappropriate care wastes valuable resources and poses legal hazards.

Quality and appropriateness indicators may be clinical, professional, or administrative. They may also be process or outcome. Figure 7-1 depicts the relationship of the various types of indicators.

Seriousness of Events. Indicators are also classified by the seriousness of the events they measure. A sentinel event measures a serious, undesirable, and often avoidable process or outcome.[4] Although the frequency is low, the event is so severe that individual case review is required. This type of indicator is described in Chapter 6.

A comparative rate or rate-based indicator measures an event that requires intensive review only if the rate of occurrence exceeds a preset threshold. These are situations for which a variance in care is allowed. For example, the number of patients with acquired stage IV dermal ulcers is a rate-based indicator because of the virtual certainty that among these patients will be an aged diabetic in end-stage renal failure associated with peripheral vascular disease, stroke, hemiplegia, and incontinence. In such a patient, it is impossible to prevent skin breakdown. Moreover, a small number of other patients will acquire dermal ulcers despite optimal nursing. The rate-based indicator acknowledges these inevitable occurrences.

Characteristics of Indicators. Olivas and coworkers describe the lack of understanding and the inability to control the care delivery process as major barriers to achieving quality.[7] The result is a failure to select appropriate variables that will forecast change, a failure to monitor these variables, and a failure to adjust activities to conform to the standards for the service.

Indicators are those forecasting variables that serve as the barometers of quality in nursing service and are the best predictors of quality or its absence. To provide meaningful information, indicators must possess five key characteristics: they must be reliable, clinically valid, measurable, specific and relevant.

Indicators must be reliable. Reliability refers to the accuracy of indicators over time, between raters, and across patients; that is, results are consistent regardless of who is collecting the data, when the data are collected, or from which source the data

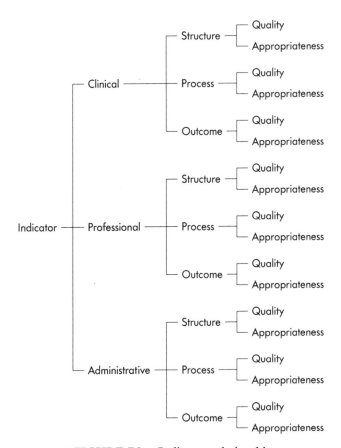

■ **FIGURE 7-1   Indicator relationships.**

are obtained. To be considered reliable, a thermometer must provide an accurate reading of body temperature regardless of which nurse is taking the temperature, what time of day the temperature is taken, or which patient's temperature is being taken. In one hospital, the reliability of the newer digital thermometers was questioned. Many nurses and physicians preferred the glass thermometers; however, there were numerous infection control and cost issues related to the use of glass thermometers. To assure staff and doctors of the accuracy of the digital thermometers, a study was done comparing the results obtained with each type. The findings confirmed the reliability of the digital thermometers in measuring body temperature, and the use of glass thermometers was abandoned.

Clinical indicators need to be reliable. The practitioner using them has to feel confident in their ability to measure the variables that they are designed to measure, regardless of who is collecting the data, when, or from which patient. The indicators that measure the number of dermal ulcers ensure that there is a consistent and accurate means by which dermal ulcers are staged. The use of a standard tool such as the Norton scale provides that assurance.

Indicators must be accurate and valid. Just because a tool is reliable does not necessarily mean that it is valid. You would not use a meat thermometer to measure a patient's temperature; nor would you use a patient satisfaction survey to measure the outcomes of diabetes teaching.

A valid tool measures what it is designed to measure.[9] For example, a thermometer measures temperature; it cannot be used to measure blood pressure.

A valid indicator identifies situations in which quality is lacking, e.g., that the number of nosocomial infections is on the rise or that the number of unsupported patient falls resulting in injury is escalating. A valid indicator would identify that nurses are not turning high-risk patients every 2 hours or that diabetic patients remain unable to recognize the signs and symptoms of hypoglycemia and intervene appropriately even after instruction.

Indicators must be measurable. The promotion of a safe environment is not a measurable indicator, whereas the number of unsupported patient falls not involving injury is. You cannot manage what you cannot measure.[1] Important aspects of service must be translated into measurable, quantifiable variables.

Indicators must be specific and definite. Specificity relates to the precision with which the indicator measures the event. Indicators must apply to, characterize, or denote a particular issue or event. They are an exact written description of a specification. For example, an indicator related to chemotherapy is specific to cancer patients, while an indicator related to fetal monitoring characterizes care given only to obstetric patients.

Indicators must be relevant to patients, to staff, and to the system. They should focus on the critical aspects of the service, not the marginal issues, and touch on every subsystem of the care process. For example, on a surgical unit, indicators should relate to preoperative preparation and postoperative recovery.

■ THE INDICATOR INFORMATION SET

The Joint Commission recommends completing the following information before using an indicator: definition of terms, indicator type, rationale for use of the indicator, description of the indicator population, indicator data collection logic, and delineation of underlying factors that may explain variations in indicator data. This information is termed an indicator information set.[8]

Defining the terms used in the indicator ensures that everyone using the indicator is monitoring the same data. Uniform operational definitions ensure uniform understanding.

Identification of indicator type means differentiating between a rate-based event versus a sentinel event or a process verses an outcome, while the rationale defines how or why the indicator will be beneficial. "By stating the rationale for an indicator, those considering the indicator gain a deeper understanding of its potential value and can better judge its merits."[8]

Description of the indicator population includes those patient groups for which the indicator is relevant. For example, an indicator may be developed to measure patients who sustain a fall and have a serious injury within 2 hours of sedative administration. The indicator population may be composed of those patients receiving sedatives. Subcategories add specificity to the indicator population. For example, the subcategories of patients over the age of 75 years or ambulatory surgical patients provide homogeneous populations to be assessed. Because different circumstances are at play for these populations, it is important to pinpoint specific populations so that the appropriate improvement strategies can be designed.

Indicator data logic refers to the development of data elements. Data elements are used to define the indicator event. "Terms used in the indicator are translated into specific data elements, and corresponding data sources are identified by which data elements may be retrieved."[8] Data elements associated with the falls indicator might include the time elapsed between the administration of the sedative and the fall and the type of sedative administered. It is from the data sources that specific information about the data elements is obtained. For example, review of the patient's progress record and the medication administration record would reveal the interval between the sedative administration and the fall. The type of sedative administered would be obtained from the physician's order sheet or the medication administration record.

Delineation of potential underlying factors refers to the identification of specific patient, practitioner, or system variables related to the indicator which have a direct impact on the quality of patient outcomes for that important aspect of care. Patient variables include severity of illness, comorbid conditions, and any other nondisease factors that may affect the frequency of the event occurrence. Nondisease factors may include patient demographics. Patient variables may be beyond the control of the staff or system. Practitioner variables are those conditions related to the practitioner's performance that may potentially affect the quality of patient outcomes vis à vis an important aspect of care. These factors usually relate to the practitioner's competence or productivity. System variables are those factors within the system that directly affect the quality of care provided and thus the patient outcomes for a particular aspect of care. The factors can include staffing, budgeting, or equipment availability. Unlike patient variables, both practitioner and system variables can be controlled.

■ THE JOINT COMMISSION'S DEVELOPMENT OF INDICATORS

In the fall of 1986, the Joint Commission launched a major initiative called the Agenda for Change. The project was implemented to improve the Joint Commission's ability to evaluate the clinical and organizational performance of health care organizations. Its goal is to develop an outcome-focused monitoring and evaluation process that will assist the organizations in improving the quality of care they provide.

Developing Clinical Indicators

One of the chief aspects of this developmental program is the design and testing of clinical indicators that relate to important aspects of care. These indicators will be used to monitor diagnostic and treatment activities relevant to the processes and outcomes of that care. It is projected that information related to these indicators will be pooled, and the institution as well as patients and third party payers will be able to compare the institution's results to those of comparable institutions. It will be similar to the comparisons made in other industries. For example, in the airline industry, comparisons are made of the on-time arrival record or the frequency and volume of luggage being lost.

Initially, three areas were chosen for indicator development. Task forces were assigned to study obstetrics, anesthesia, and hospital-wide care. The task force members and the Joint Commission project specialists soon found that the literature provided little assistance in defining indicators because of the virtual absence of professional consensus. Eventually, however, 48 indicators were developed in the three areas and pilot tested in 17 hospitals across the country.

The purpose of the testing was to identify and assess problems in data collection and to improve the efficiency of the process for data collection. Refinement or abandonment of the initial indicators was contingent on the feedback from the pilot sites.

Initially there were 70 areas for hospital-wide indicator development. These were condensed in seven major groups: mortality; medication errors; complications and unanticipated procedures related to surgery and other procedures; readmission within 30 days of scheduled surgery; hospital-acquired decubitus ulcers; nosocomial infections; and assessment of antibiotic therapy. Feedback from the pilot sites sent the Joint Commission Task Force "back to the drawing board," because many of these initial indicators did not apply hospital-wide but were more specialty specific. For example, proper timing of antibiotic prophylaxis for specified surgical procedures had no relevance for medical units. Likewise, development of pneumonia in patients treated in special care units by definition applied only to critical care.

Two areas were defined as "key functions" in hospital care. These are the appropriate and effective use of medications and the prevention, detection, and control of infections. These functions involve more than one department within the hospital; their results depend on the performance of clinical management and support services. The role of specific disciplines in each of these key functions is being outlined through task analysis. For example, nursing, medicine, pharmacy, and clerical staff play a role in medication administration. A task analysis would reveal the relevant activities of each discipline and the relationship among them.[2]

Task forces have been assembled to develop indicators on the key functions of medication use and infection control. The medication use task force held its first meeting in March, 1989. Initially, a flow chart was developed to outline key tasks and the relationships among specific disciplines and departments (see Figure 7-2). Indicators will then be developed based on the key processes. Thirteen potential target areas for indicator development were identified. Recommended key processes for measurement include:

Correct drug selection
Dosage individualization for the patient
Drug preparation
Medication administration to the right patient
Patient education about medications

**Key Function: Appropriate, Safe, Effective, and
Efficient Use of Medications**

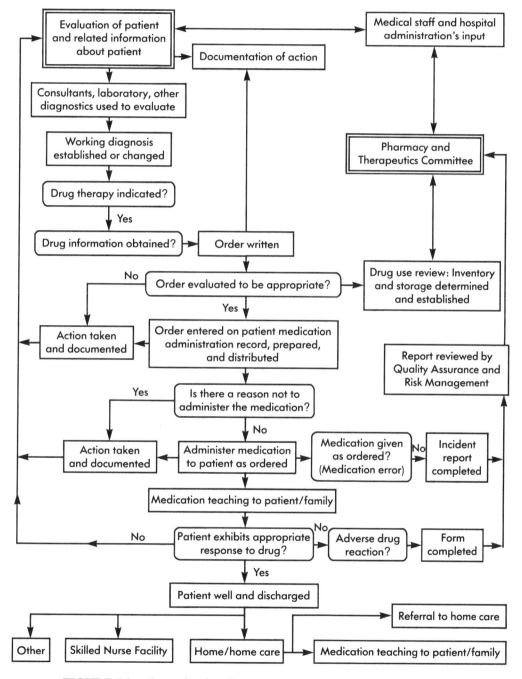

■ **FIGURE 7-2** **Example of medication usage flow diagram.** (Copyright 1990
by the Joint Commission on Accreditation of Healthcare Organizations, Oakbrook Terrace, IL.
Reprinted from Primer on indicator development and application, with permission.)

MEDICATION USE INDICATORS FOR ALPHA TESTING: SUMMARY LIST

MU-1

INDICATOR FOCUS: Individualizing dosage
Indicator (Numerator): Inpatients over 65 years old in whom creatinine clearance has been estimated.

MU-2

INDICATOR FOCUS: Individualizing dosage
Indicator (Numerator): Inpatients under 1 year old receiving parenteral aminoglycosides who have a measured aminoglycoside serum level.

MU-3

INDICATOR FOCUS: Reviewing the order
Indicator (Numerator): New medication orders prompting consultation by the pharmacist with physician or nurse subcategorized by orders changed.

MU-4

INDICATOR FOCUS: Timing of medication administration
Indicator (Numerator): Inpatients receiving intravenous prophylactic antibiotics within 2 hours before the first surgical incision.

MU-5

INDICATOR FOCUS: Accuracy of medication dispensing and administration
Indicator (Numerator): Number of reported significant medication errors.

MU-6

INDICATOR FOCUS: Informing the patient about the medication
Indicator (Numerator): Inpatients with principal and/or other diagnoses of insulin-dependent diabetes mellitus who demonstrate self blood glucose monitoring and self-administration of insulin before discharge, subcategorized by referral for postdischarge evaluation.

MU-7

INDICATOR FOCUS: Monitoring patient response
Indicator (Numerator): Inpatients receiving digoxin, theophylline, phenytoin, or lithium who have no corresponding measured drug levels or whose highest measured level exceeds a specific limit.

MU-8

INDICATOR FOCUS: Monitoring patient response
Indicator (Numerator): Inpatients over 65 years old receiving tricyclic antidepressants who fall.

MEDICATION USE INDICATORS FOR ALPHA TESTING: SUMMARY LIST—cont'd

MU-9

INDICATOR FOCUS: Monitoring patient response
Indicator (Numerator): Inpatients receiving anticoagulant therapy who also receive Vitamin K, protamine sulfate, or fresh frozen plasma, subcategorized by ADRs reported to the ADR reporting system for the patients above.

MU-10

INDICATOR FOCUS: Reporting adverse drug reactions
Indicator (Numerator): ADRs reported through the hospital's ADR reporting system subcategorized by method of reporting (concurrent or retrospective medical record abstraction) and by type of ADR (dose related or non-dose related).

MU-11

INDICATOR FOCUS: Reviewing complete therapeutic drug regimen
Indicator (Numerator): Inpatients receiving more than one type of benzodiazepine simultaneously.

MU-12

INDICATOR FOCUS: Reviewing complete therapeutic drug regimen
Indicator (Numerator): Inpatients with seven or more prescribed medications on discharge.

MU-13

INDICATOR FOCUS: System/management control
Indicator (Numerator): Inpatients who have an allergy to penicillin recorded in the medical record and who receive penicillin.

MU-14

INDICATOR FOCUS: Appropriate prescribing
Indicator (Numerator): Pediatric inpatients with febrile viral illness receiving aspirin (ASA).

MU-15

INDICATOR FOCUS: Overall performance of medication use system
Indicator (Numerator): Patients with a principal diagnosis of bronchoconstrictive pulmonary disease, who are readmitted to the hospital or visit the emergency department within 15 days of discharge due to an exacerbation of their principal diagnosis.

INFECTION CONTROL INDICATORS FOR ALPHA TESTING: SUMMARY LIST

IC-1

INDICATOR FOCUS: Surgical wound infection
Indicator (Numerator): Selected surgical operations complicated by a wound infection.

IC-2

INDICATOR FOCUS: Postpartum endometritis
Indicator (Numerator): Patients who develop endometritis within 3 postoperative days following cesarean section.

IC-3

INDICATOR FOCUS: Primary bloodstream infection
Indicator (Numerator): Patients with a central or umbilical line who develop primary bloodstream infection.

IC-4

INDICATOR FOCUS: Ventilator pneumonia
Indicator (Numerator): Ventilated patients who develop pneumonia.

IC-5

INDICATOR FOCUS: Postoperative pneumonia
Indicator (Numerator): Selected surgical operations complicated by the onset of pneumonia during hospitalization but not beyond 10 postoperative days.

IC-6

INDICATOR FOCUS: Urinary catheter usage
Indicator (Numerator): Selected surgical operations on patients who are catheterized during the perioperative period.

IC-7

INDICATOR FOCUS: Employee health program
Indicator (Numerator): Hospital employees who have been immunized for measles (rubeola) or are known to be immune.

IC-8

INDICATOR FOCUS: Surveillance/Medical Record Review
Indicator (Numerator): Patients with a central or umbilical line and primary bloodstream infection identified through both medical record review *and* surveillance activities.

The box on pp. 82-83 lists the medication use indicators in alpha testing.

The infection control task force met for the first time in January 1990. The focus of their work was nosocomial infections. The process of infection control did not readily lend itself to flowcharts. However, since nosocomial infection rates have been monitored since the 1970s, it was felt that this data base in conjunction with extensive field experience in surveillance practices would serve as a foundation for indicator development. These indicators are expected to foster better use of current data in an effort to reduce the risks of nosocomial infections.[4] The box on p. 84 lists the infection control indicators in alpha testing.

Five major aspects of care were selected as the basis for the obstetrical indicators. These include prenatal care, maternal complications, cesarean sections, neonatal complications, and obstetrical-related mortality. The box on p. 86 lists the 21 initial obstetrical indicators. Feedback from alpha testing led to revisions (see box on p. 87).

Eight important aspects of care formed the basis for the anesthesia indicators. These include anesthesia-related mortality; neurological deficits; cardiovascular complications; pulmonary complications; technical problems including mechanical trauma; protocol changes; transfusion and renal problems; and laboratory indications of anesthesia-related difficulties. The box on p. 88 lists the original 14 anesthesia indicators. The box on p. 89 lists the revised indicators that resulted from alpha testing.

Both obstetric and anesthesia indicators became available for use in 1991. Their use, however, remains optional.

New sets of indicators have been developed in cardiovascular, oncology, and trauma care. Sixty indicators that include process and outcome, appropriateness, and effectiveness have been designed. Alpha testing at new pilot sites began in 1990. Beta testing began in the spring of 1991.

Cardiovascular indicators include angioplasty, coronary artery bypass graft, myocardial infarction, and congestive heart failure. The box on pp. 90-91 lists the new cardiovascular indicators for beta testing.

The trauma indicators encompass prehospital care, emergency department care, operating room, and intensive care unit. The box on pp. 92-93 lists the trauma indicators for beta testing.

Oncology indicators focus on the three most common tumor sites in adults: breast, colorectal region, and lung. The box on pp. 94-95 lists the oncology indicators for beta testing. In October 1990, a core group met to define the function of home infusion therapy and to delineate the scope of care for indicator development. The development of home care indicators is the first project that is nonhospital based.[4] The flowchart in Figure 7-3 depicts home infusion therapy as a system. Candidate areas for further indicator development include laboratory services, imaging services, preoperative care, mental health services, long-term care, and ambulatory care.[5]

Eventually all areas of health care specialties will develop generic clinical indicators as the benchmark of quality. These indicators will ultimately drive the evaluation of hospital clinical data systems.

Performance indicators will ultimately be useful to:

Develop/refine practice guidelines
Identify alternative care delivery mechanisms/processes
Allocate resources
Foster collaborative practice
Drive quality education

Text continues on p. 95.

OBSTETRICAL CARE INDICATORS (ORIGINAL)

1. The induction of labor for indications other than diabetes, premature rupture of membranes, pregnancy-induced hypertension, post-term gestation, intrauterine growth retardation, cardiac disease, isoimmunization, fetal demise, or chorioamnionitis with or without a cesarean section.
2. A primary cesarean section for failure to progress.
3. A successful or failed vaginal birth after cesarean section (VBAC).
4. The delivery of an infant by planned repeat cesarean section weighing less than 2500 grams or with hyaline membrane disease.
5. The delivery of an infant following the induction of labor weighing less than 2500 grams or with hyaline membrane disease.
6. Eclampsia.
7. The in-hospital initiation of antibiotics 24 hours or more after a term vaginal delivery.
8. Excessive maternal blood loss except with abruptio placenta or placenta previa as evidenced by either a red cell transfusion, a hematocrit less than 22 or a hemoglobin less than 7, or a decrease in hematocrit of more than 11 or of hemoglobin more than 3.5.
9. A maternal length of stay more than 5 days after a vaginal delivery or more than 7 days after a cesarean section.
10. A maternal readmission within 14 days of delivery.
11. A maternal death up to and including 42 days postpartum.
12. The in-hospital intrapartum death of a fetus weighing 500 grams or more.
13. The perinatal death of an infant weighing 500 grams or more.
14. The neonatal death of an infant with a birth weight of 750-999 grams born in a hospital with a NICU.
15. The delivery of an infant weighing less than 1800 grams in a hospital without a NICU.
16. The transfer of a neonate to a NICU at another hospital.
17. A term infant admitted to a NICU.
18. An Apgar score of 3 or less at 5 minutes.
19. The diagnosis of massive aspiration syndrome referenced as ICD9-CM code 770.1.
20. The diagnosis of birth trauma referenced as ICD-9-CM code 767.
21. A term infant having a clinically apparent seizure prior to discharge from the delivery hospital.

From Joint Commission on Accreditation of Healthcare Organizations, Agenda for Change UPDATE 2(1), June 1988. Used with permission.

OBSTETRICAL CARE INDICATORS (REVISED)

1. Patients with primary cesarean section for failure to progress.
2. Patients with attempted vaginal birth after cesarean section (VBAC), subcategorized by success or failure.
3. Patients with excessive maternal blood loss defined by either post-delivery red blood cell transfusion or a low post-delivery hematocrit or hemoglobin (Hct < 22%, Hgb < 7 gms) or a significant pre- to post-delivery decrease in hematocrit (decrease ≥ 11%) or hemoglobin (decrease ≥ 3.5 gms) excluding patients with abruptio placenta or placenta previa.
4. Patients with diagnosis of eclampsia.
5. The delivery of infants weighing less than 2500 grams, following either induction of labor or repeat cesarean section without medical indications.*
6. Term infants admitted to a neonatal intensive care unit (NICU) within 24 hours of delivery and with NICU stay greater than 24 hours excluding admissions for major congenital anomalies.*
7. Neonates with an Apgar score of 3 or less at 5 minutes and a birthweight greater than 1500 grams.
8. Neonates with a discharge diagnosis of significant birth trauma.*
9. Term infants with a diagnosis of hypoxic encephalopathy or clinically apparent seizure prior to discharge from the hospital of birth, excluding newborns with a diagnosis of fetal alcohol syndrome, and other drug reactions and withdrawal syndromes.
10. Deaths of infants weighing 500 grams or more subcategorized by intrahospital neonatal deaths, total stillborns and intrapartum stillborns.

Reprinted with permission of Joint Commission on Accreditation of Healthcare Organizations.
*A list of the specific diagnoses and appropriate ICD-9-CM diagnostic codes for medical indications for induction of labor and repeat cesareans, for major congenital anomalies, and for significant birth trauma will be provided with the data element specifications for the obstetrics indicators.

ANESTHESIA CARE INDICATORS (ORIGINAL)

1. Mortality within a specified time* following anesthesia care.
2. Failure to emerge from general anesthesia within a specified time.
3. Development of injury to the brain or spinal cord within a specified time following anesthesia care.
4. Development of a peripheral neurologic deficit within a specified time following anesthesia care.
5. Cardiac arrest within a specified time following anesthesia care.
6. Clinically apparent acute myocardial infarction within a specified time following anesthesia care.
7. Fulminant pulmonary edema within a specified time following anesthesia care.
8. Respiratory arrest within a specified time following anesthesia care.
9. Aspiration of gastric contents with development of typical x-ray findings of aspiration pneumonitis within a specified time following anesthesia care.
10. Development of postdural puncture headache within a specified time following anesthesia care.
11. Dental injury during anesthesia care.
12. Ocular injury during anesthesia care.
13. Unplanned hospital admission within a specified time following an outpatient procedure involving anesthesia.
14. Unplanned admission to an intensive care unit within a specified time following administration of an anesthetic.

From Joint Commission on Accreditation of Healthcare Organizations, Agenda for Change UPDATE 2(1), June 1988. Used with permission.

*All time ranges will be specified following evaluation and analysis of pilot-site empirical data.

ANESTHESIA CARE INDICATORS SUMMARY LIST

1. Patients developing a CNS complication occurring during or within 2 post-procedure days of procedures involving anesthesia administration, subcategorized by ASA-PS class, patient age, and CNS vs. non–CNS related procedures.
2. Patients developing a peripheral neurologic deficit during or within 2 post-procedure days of procedures involving anesthesia administration.
3. Patients developing an acute myocardial infarction during or within 2 post-procedure days of procedures involving anesthesia administration, subcategorized by ASA-PS class, patient age, and cardiac vs. noncardiac procedures.
4. Patients with a cardiac arrest during or within 1 postprocedure day of procedures involving anesthesia administration, excluding patients with required intraoperative cardiac arrest, subcategorized by ASA-PS class, patient age, and cardiac vs. noncardiac procedures.
5. Patients with unplanned respiratory arrest during or within 1 postprocedure day of procedures involving anesthesia administration.
6. Death of patients during or within 2 postprocedure days of procedures involving anesthesia administration, subcategorized by ASA-PS class and patient age.
7. Unplanned admission of patients to the hospital within 1 postprocedure day following outpatient procedures involving anesthesia administration.
8. Unplanned admission of patients to an intensive care unit within 1 postprocedure day of procedures involving anesthesia administration and with ICU stay greater than 1 day.

Reprinted with permission of Joint Commission on Accreditation of Healthcare Organizations.

CARDIOVASCULAR INDICATORS FOR BETA TESTING

Cardiovascular Indicator Patient Population: The Cardiovascular indicators draw from four populations described below: CABG, PTCA, AMI, and CHF.

CABG Patient Population: Patients undergoing coronary artery bypass grafts (CABG) excluding those with other cardiac or peripheral vascular surgical procedures performed at the time of the CABG (e.g., valve replacement).

CV-1

INDICATOR FOCUS: Intrahospital mortality as a means of assessing multiple aspects of CABG care
Indicator (Numerator): Intrahospital mortality of patients undergoing isolated coronary artery bypass graft (CABG) procedures, subcategorized by initial and subsequent CABG procedures, by emergent or nonemergent clinical status, and by postoperative day and intrahospital location of death.

CV-2

INDICATOR FOCUS: Extended postoperative stay as a means of assessing multiple aspects of CABG care.
Indicator (Numerator): Patients with prolonged postoperative stay for isolated coronary artery bypass graft (CABG) procedures, subcategorized by initial or subsequent CABG procedures, by emergent or nonemergent procedures, and by the use or nonuse of a circulatory support device.

PTCA Patient Population: Patients for whom a percutaneous transluminal coronary angioplasty (PTCA) procedure is initiated, regardless of whether or not a lesion is crossed or dilated.

CV-3

INDICATOR FOCUS: Intrahospital mortality as a means of assessing multiple aspects of PTCA care
Indicator (Numerator): Intrahospital mortality of patients following percutaneous transluminal coronary angioplasty (PTCA), subcategorized by emergent or nonemergent clinical status and by postprocedure day and intrahospital location of death.

CV-4

INDICATOR FOCUS: Specific clinical events as a means of assessing multiple aspects of PTCA care
Indicator (Numerator): Patients undergoing nonemergent percutaneous transluminal coronary angioplasty (PTCA) with subsequent occurrence of either an acute myocardial infarction (MI) or coronary artery bypass graft (CABG) procedure within the same hospitalization.

Reprinted with permission of Joint Commission on Accreditation of Healthcare Organizations.

CARDIOVASCULAR INDICATORS FOR BETA TESTING— cont'd

CV-5

INDICATOR FOCUS: Effectiveness of PTCA
Indicator (Numerator): Patients undergoing attempted or completed percutaneous transluminal coronary angioplasty (PTCA) during which any lesion attempted is not dilated.

MI Patient Population: Patients with a principal diagnosis of acute myocardial infarction (MI) either upon hospital discharge, emergency department (ED) transfer to another acute care facility, or death in the emergency department (ED), and patients who are admitted for an acute MI or to rule out an acute MI.

CV-6

INDICATOR FOCUS: Intrahospital mortality as a means of assessing multiple aspects of acute MI care
Indicator (Numerator): Intrahospital mortality of patients with principal discharge diagnosis of acute myocardial infarction (MI), subcategorized by history of previous infarction, age, and intrahospital location of death.

CV-7

INDICATOR FOCUS: Diagnostic accuracy and resource utilization
Indicator (Numerator): Patients admitted for acute myocardial infarction (MI), rule-out acute MI, or unstable angina who have a discharge diagnosis of acute MI, subcategorized by admission to an intensive care unit, a monitored bed, or an unmonitored bed.

CHF Patient Population: Patients with a principal discharge diagnosis of congestive heart failure, with or without specific etiologies.

CV-8

INDICATOR FOCUS: Diagnostic accuracy
Indicator (Numerator): Patients with principal discharge diagnosis of congestive heart failure (CHF) with documented etiology and chest X-ray substantiation of CHF.

CV-9

INDICATOR FOCUS: Monitoring patient's response to therapy
Indicator (Numerator): Patients with a principal discharge diagnosis of congestive heart failure (CHF) and with at least two determinations of patient weight and of serum sodium, potassium, blood urea nitrogen (BUN), and creatinine levels.

TRAUMA INDICATORS FOR BETA TESTING

Trauma Patient Population: Patients with ICD-9-CM diagnostic code of 800 through 959.9 who are either admitted to the hospital, die in the emergency department (ED), or transferred from the hospital or the ED to another acute care facility, excluding patients with the following isolated injuries: burns; hip fractures in the elderly; specified fractures of the face, hand, and foot; and specified eye wounds.

TR-1

INDICATOR FOCUS: Efficiency of emergency medical services (EMS)
Indicator (Numerator): Trauma patients with prehospital emergency medical services (EMS) scene time greater than 20 minutes.

TR-2

INDICATOR FOCUS: Ongoing monitoring of trauma patients
Indicator (Numerator): Trauma patients with blood pressure, pulse, respiration, and Glasgow Coma Scale (GCS) documented in the emergency department (ED) record on arrival and hourly until inpatient admission to operating room or intensive care unit, death, or transfer to another care facility (hourly GCS needed only if altered state of consciousness).

TR-3

INDICATOR FOCUS: Airway management of comatose trauma patients
Indicator (Numerator): Comatose patients discharged from the emergency department (ED) prior to the establishment of a mechanical airway.

TR-4

INDICATOR FOCUS: Timeliness of diagnostic testing
Indicator (Numerator): Trauma patients with diagnosis of intracranial injury and altered state of consciousness upon emergency department (ED) arrival receiving initial head computerized tomography (CT) scan greater than 2 hours after ED arrival.

TR-5

INDICATOR FOCUS: Timeliness of surgical intervention for adult head injury
Indicator (Numerator): Trauma patients with diagnosis of extradural or subdural brain hemorrhage undergoing craniotomy greater than 4 hours after emergency department (ED) arrival (excluding intracranial pressure monitoring), subcategorized by pediatric or adult patients.

TR-6

INDICATOR FOCUS: Timeliness of surgical intervention for orthopedic injuries
Indicator (Numerator): Trauma patients with open fractures of the long bones as a result of blunt trauma receiving initial surgical treatment greater than 8 hours after emergency department (ED) arrival.

Reprinted with permission of Joint Commission on Accreditation of Healthcare Organizations.

TRAUMA INDICATORS FOR BETA TESTING—cont'd

TR-7

INDICATOR FOCUS: Timeliness of surgical intervention for abdominal injuries
Indicator (Numerator): Trauma patients with diagnosis of laceration of the liver or spleen, requiring surgery, undergoing laparotomy greater than 2 hours after emergency department (ED) arrival, subcategorized by pediatric or adult patients.

TR-8

INDICATOR FOCUS: Surgical decision making for abdominal gunshot wounds versus stab wounds
Indicator (Numerator): Trauma patients undergoing laparotomy for wounds penetrating the abdominal wall, subcategorized by gunshot versus stab wounds.

TR-9

INDICATOR FOCUS: Timeliness of patient transfers
Indicator (Numerator): Trauma patients transferred from initial receiving hospital to another acute care facility within 6 hours from emergency department (ED) arrival to ED departure.

TR-10

INDICATOR FOCUS: Surgical decision making for orthopedic injuries
Indicator (Numerator): Adult trauma patients with femoral diaphyseal fractures treated by a non-fixation technique.

TR-11

INDICATOR FOCUS: Clinical decision making for potentially preventable deaths
Indicator (Numerator): Intrahospital mortality of trauma patients with one or more of the following conditions who did not undergo a procedure for the condition: tension pneumothorax, hemoperitoneum, hemothoraces, ruptured aorta, pericardial tamponade, and epidural or subdural hemorrhage.

TR-12

INDICATOR FOCUS: Systems necessary for obtaining autopsies for trauma victims
Indicator (Numerator): Trauma patients who expired within 48 hours of emergency department (ED) arrival for whom an autopsy was performed.

ONCOLOGY INDICATORS FOR BETA TESTING

Oncology Patient Population: Inpatients admitted for initial diagnosis and/or treatment of primary lung, colon, rectal, or female breast cancer.

ON-1

INDICATOR FOCUS: Availability of data for diagnosis and staging
Indicator (Numerator): Surgical pathology consultation reports (pathology reports) containing histological type, tumor size, status of margins, appropriate lymph node examination, assessment of invasion or extension as indicated, and AJCC/pTN classification for patients with resection for primary cancer of the lung, colon/rectum, or female breast.

ON-2

INDICATOR FOCUS: Use of staging by managing physicians
Indicator (Numerator): Patients undergoing treatment for primary cancer of the lung, colon/rectum, or female breast with AJCC stage of tumor designated by a managing physician.

ON-3

INDICATOR FOCUS: Effectiveness of cancer treatment
Indicator (Numerator): Survival of patients with primary cancer of the lung, colon/rectum, or female breast by stage and histologic type.*

ON-4

INDICATOR FOCUS: Use of tests critical to diagnosis, prognosis, and clinical management
Indicator (Numerator): Female patients with invasive primary breast cancer undergoing initial biopsy or resection of a tumor larger than 1 cm in greatest dimension who have presence of estrogen receptor diagnostic analysis results in medical record.

ON-5

INDICATOR FOCUS: Use of multimodal therapy in treatment and follow-up
Indicator (Numerator): Female patients with AJCC Stage II pathologic lymph node positive primary invasive breast cancer treated with systemic adjuvant therapy.

ON-6

INDICATOR FOCUS: Effectiveness of preoperative diagnosis and staging
Indicator (Numerator): Patients with non-small cell primary lung cancer undergoing thoracotomy with complete surgical resection of tumor.

ON-7

INDICATOR FOCUS: Specific clinical events as a means of assessing multiple aspects of surgical care for lung cancers
Indicator (Numerator): Patients undergoing pulmonary resection for primary lung cancer with postoperative complication of empyema, bronchopleural fistula, reoperation for postoperative bleeding, mechanical ventilation greater than 5 days postop, or intrahospital death.

Reprinted with permission of Joint Commission on Accreditation of Healthcare Organizations.
*Efficient mechanisms to obtain postdischarge data will be explored only with a subset of Beta test hospitals. Ability to obtain this data during Beta testing is not a requirement for participation.

ONCOLOGY INDICATORS FOR BETA TESTING—cont'd

ON-8

INDICATOR FOCUS: Comprehensiveness of diagnostic workup
Indicator (Numerator): Patients with resections of primary colorectal cancer whose preoperative evaluation by a managing physician includes examination of the entire colon, liver function tests, chest x-ray, and carcinoembryonic antigen (CEA) levels.

ON-9

INDICATOR FOCUS: Documentation of staging, prognosis, and surgical treatment
Indicator (Numerator): Patients with resection of primary colorectal cancer whose operative reports include location of primary tumor, local extent of disease, extent of resection, and assessment of residual abdominal disease.

ON-10

INDICATOR FOCUS: Use of treatment approaches which impact on quality of life
Indicator (Numerator): Patients with primary rectal cancer undergoing abdominoperineal resections with 6 cm or more of free distal surgical margin present on specimen, as documented in surgical pathology gross description.

ON-11

INDICATOR FOCUS: Interdisciplinary treatment and follow-up
Indicator (Numerator): Patients with AJCC Stage II or III primary rectal cancer with documentation of referral to or treatment by a radiation or medical oncologist.

■ DEVELOPING ORGANIZATIONAL INDICATORS

Along with the clinical indicators, the Joint Commission determined that there must be mechanisms to ensure that the organization is able to facilitate the delivery of quality care. "Since management effectiveness is one of the prerequisites for improving an organization's clinical performance, the Joint Commission set out to identify those principles of organizational and management effectiveness that could be used to guide standards revision as well as indicator development."[3] These principles focus on innovative leadership, system-wide assessment based on feedback from internal and external customers or users of the institution's services, and total organizational commitment to continuous improvement in quality of care.

Organizational indicators are being developed related to the leadership functions and those that address support and operations. They demonstrate the organization's commitment to continual improvement. The box on p. 97 lists the 12 principles upon which indicators will be developed. These indicators will help an institution to analyze objectively how their organization and management affect the quality of care provided. These principles emphasize the following points:

- The organization—not its individual units—is accountable for quality of care.
- Commitment to continual improvement should be pervasive in day-to-day organizational function.

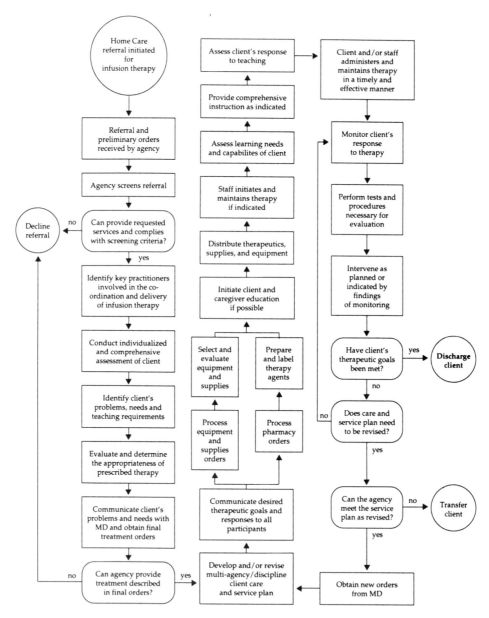

■ **FIGURE 7-3** **Infusion therapy in the home care setting.**
(Copyright 1991 by the Joint Commission on Accreditation of Healthcare Organizations,
Oakbrook Terrace, IL. Reprinted with permission from the March/April 1991
Joint Commission Perspectives.)

PRINCIPLES OF ORGANIZATIONAL AND MANAGEMENT EFFECTIVENESS

- Mission
- Culture
- Strategic, program, and research plans
- Organizational change
- Role of governing body and management and clinical leadership
- Leadership qualifications, development, and assessment
- Resources
- Clinical competence of independent practitioners
- Recruitment, development, evaluation, and retention policies and practices
- Evaluation and improvement of patient care
- Organizational integration and coordination
- Continuity and comprehensiveness of care

From Joint Commission on Accreditation of Healthcare Organizations, Agenda for Change UPDATE 2(1), June 1988. Used with permission.

- Effective internal coordination and collaboration among governance, management, practitioners, and other staff are essential to the support of quality improvement activities.
- The payoff is performance. Structural requirements should largely be an organizational prerogative and should be designed to support organizational performance objectives.
- Performance must be rigorously monitored through the application of effective measures that examine clinical care, management, and vital internal processes.[6]

■ COLLABORATIVE QUALITY ASSESSMENT

The work of the Joint Commission has given rise to much anxiety and confusion in the minds of nurses throughout the country. Many of the indicators that have been developed to date seem to focus on medical outcomes. Is the Joint Commission saying that we must monitor only these outcomes? If so, how can nursing monitor medical outcomes? Do we need to change the thrust of our monitoring plans?

"The Joint Commission has neither the desire nor the intent to be the sole or even the primary source for indicator development. Indeed, health care organizations must themselves eventually determine the unique aspects of the services they provide and develop appropriate additional measures to monitor performance."[3]

Traditionally, quality assurance has been categorized by discipline. Redundancy in monitoring can occur across disciplines if both nursing and medicine or services such as social work or respiratory therapy monitor the same parameters. However, the data collected by each discipline are also less useful if not fully integrated. Collaborative quality assessment is the ideal. Indicators are developed within each discipline based on its contribution to the desired patient outcome for a particular patient problem or symptomatology. For example, nurses, physicians, social workers, and respiratory therapists all care for acutely ill COPD patients. They all address the problem of impaired gas exchange. The physician orders medications, the nurse administers postural drainage, the respiratory therapist coordinates the oxygen therapy, and the social worker makes arrangements for home oxygen therapy. Improved patient outcome is contingent on all of the disciplines working together to correct the problem. The general outcome indicator would reflect correction of the impaired gas exchange and each discipline would focus its monitoring on those activities and specific outcomes that contribute to the desired overall outcome. The focus of collaborative quality assessment is on the patient rather than on the discipline, as had been the case.

This collaborative approach also is effective when the problem is organizational or professional. For example, medication administration involves physicians who order the drugs, pharmacists who prepare them, and nurses who administer them. Similarly, staffing involves nursing, payroll, and personnel.

■ LINKING STANDARDS AND INDICATORS

The authors believe that the generic indicators developed by the Joint Commission Task Forces will serve as umbrella indicators. Each discipline will then be responsible for evaluating its contribution to the process or outcome and designating subindicators for internal monitoring. For example, one obstetrical indicator is primary cesarean section for failure to progress in labor. While nursing does not make the ultimate decision regarding the necessity of the cesarean section, nursing does participate significantly in the ultimate outcome because of the nursing interventions aimed at facilitating progress in labor. Nursing may identify specific patient outcomes related to labor progress such as:

- Three contractions within a 10-minute period. For the internally monitored patient: contractions over 55 mm of pressure and 5 to 15 mm resting tone
- For the externally monitored patient: firm contractions lasting 45 to 60 seconds
- Absence of complications/emergencies

Then, practice guidelines would be developed to outline the nursing process necessary to achieve those outcomes. Nursing would then select process or outcome indicators from the standards written for that particular patient situation.

Development or worsening of pressure ulcers is another clinical indicator. Nursing plays a significant role in this outcome. However, it is not sufficient merely to record the numbers of pressure ulcers that develop. As we have seen in the past, volume indicators alone do not provide enough information to pinpoint problems or improve care. Nursing must translate that general indicator into specific nursing standards related to pressure ulcer care. These might include practice guidelines for the management of altered skin integrity: pressure ulcers and procedures for the application of special dressings or the use of special beds. Figure 7-4 is an example of a practice guideline for patients with alterations in skin integrity.

■ DEVELOPING GOOD INDICATORS

Well-developed written standards are the key to good indicators. If standards are reliable, valid, measurable, specific, and relevant, then indicators will be also. For instance, well-developed practice guidelines for the management of failure to progress in labor will define the desired outcomes and the nursing process necessary to achieve those results (Figure 7-5). Outcome or process indicators can be chosen from the information provided in that standard. The stated outcomes can be translated directly

Text continues on p. 104.

PERSONNEL

This practice guideline is divided into seven major sections. Each section may be performed as indicated.

1. Assessment: RN
2. Planning:
       In-house: RN
       Discharge: RN, LPN
3. Interventions: RN, LPN, Student Nurse, NA
4. Evaluation: RN, LPN, Student Nurse
5. Teaching: RN, LPN, Student Nurse
6. Complications: RN, LPN
7. Documentation: RN, LPN, Student Nurse

COMPETENCIES:

1. Must be documented by the education department record that employee has received inservice on pressure ulcer practice guidelines.
2. Must have passed in-house certification test in staging pressure ulcers, use of the hospital pressure ulcer sizing scale, and identification of high-risk patients.
3. Must have completed associated complicated wound management certification established by the department.

PATIENT OUTCOME:

1. The patient will maintain or improve skin integrity during length of stay.

STAFF OUTCOME:

1. Nursing personnel will identify those patients with potential for alterations in skin integrity and will institute preventive measures in a planned, organized, systematic manner throughout the institution.
2. Nursing personnel will identify those patients with actual alterations in skin integrity and institute corrective measures in a planned, organized, systematic manner.

SYSTEM OUTCOME:

1. Staffing will be maintained according to acuity ratios on all patients with actual alternations in skin integrity.
2. The subject of skin integrity will be part of every new employee orientation within the division of nursing.

INDICATIONS FOR IMPLEMENTING PRESSURE ULCER PRACTICE GUIDELINES:

1. Elderly, age 75 and over
2. Extremely thin or obese
3. Bed- or chair-fast patients, decreased mobility
4. Altered nutritional status
5. Incontinent of urine or stool
6. Preexisting lesions or history of pressure ulcers
7. Chronic illnesses affecting tissue perfusion (diabetes, peripheral vascular disease, cancer, etc.)
8. External devices (casts, traction)

INDICATIONS FOR USE OF SPECIALTY BEDS:

1. Patient unable to move or turn
2. Pressure ulcers on two or more areas
3. Evaluation by the Skin Care Team

INDICATIONS FOR STAGING PRESSURE ULCERS:

1. PREVENTIVE: At risk but no visible evidence of ulcer.
2. STAGE ONE: Redness and/or mottling that does not resolve within 30 minutes. Skin intact.
3. STAGE TWO: Skin is blistered or broken at epidermis.
4. STAGE THREE: Open area extending beyond epidermis to subcutaneous tissue with or without necrosis. May be covered with eschar.
5. STAGE FOUR: Deep open area exposing muscle, fascia, or bone. Crater may be covered with eschar.

■ **FIGURE 7-4   Practice guidelines for patients with alterations in skin integrity.**
(From Decubitus 4(1):38-42, 1991. Used with permission.)

Continued.

AREA OF RESPONSIBILITY	INTERVENTIONS
1. ASSESSMENT	1.1 Observe and inspect skin at initial assessment and every shift. Observation and inspection include: • Skin color • Ulcer size • Pain at site • Odor • Pulse • Drainage • Temperature • Blisters • Location • Condition of surrounding skin
2. PLANNING IN-HOUSE	2.1 Orient the patient to practice guidelines for alterations in skin integrity 2.2 Set goals for skin integrity 2.3 Chart and report observations to MD and Skin Care Team 2.4 Discuss specific evaluations of fluid and nutritional status with the Skin Care Team 2.5 Initiate the Pressure Ulcer Flow Sheet • Stage the skin integrity • Establish turning schedule • Institute measures to reduce shearing/friction 2.6 Determine need for pressure reduction support systems 2.7 Obtain wound culture if signs of systemic infection are present, e.g., redness, induration, fever or edema 2.8 Institute measures to reduce excessive moisture
DISCHARGE:	2.9 See TEACHING/INFORMATION SECTION 5 2.10 Arrange for home health follow-up visit if appropriate
3. INTERVENTION: PREVENTIVE:	3.1 Encourage activity: If possible, assist patient to ambulate once per day and evening shift 3.2 Place pressure reduction mattress on patient's bed. (You need a standing order or an MD order for reimbursement purposes) NOTE: DO NOT RUB RED BONY PROMINENCES!
STAGE ONE:	3.3 Institute all interventions in PREVENTIVE STAGE 3.4 Get patients OOB at least once per 24-hour period for minimum of one half hour 3.5 Turn patients every 2 hours 3.6 Utilize draw sheets at all times when moving patients 3.7 Use heel protectors on patients when in bed if heels are red 3.8 Use elbow protectors on patients in bed if their elbows are red
STAGE TWO:	3.9 Institute all interventions in PREVENTIVE STAGE AND STAGE ONE 3.10 Use normal saline for cleansing, patting rather than rubbing dry 3.11 Use transparent dressing if needed • See procedure for application and changing of pressure ulcer dressings • Change transparent dressing every 72 hours or PRN if leaking
STAGE THREE:	3.12 Institute ALL previous interventions 3.13 Discuss with the Skin Care Team the options to use other pressure reduction support surfaces 3.14 For clean, granulating, healthy, non-infected wound base, clean with normal saline 3.15 If necrotic tissue (slough or eschar) is present, clean with approved cleansing agent 3.16 Dress ulcers on all body areas EXCEPT coccyx and hip using transparent dressing (Examples: Opsite, Tegaderm, Accuderm)

■ **FIGURE 7-4, cont'd.**

AREA OF RESPONSIBILITY	INTERVENTIONS
	3.17 Dress ulcers on coccyx and hip using hydroactive wafers (Example: Duoderm CGF, Restore) • Change transparent dressing every 72 hours or PRN if leaking
	3.18 If slough or eschar are present, cover with a thin film transparent dressing to prepare the wound for debriding
	3.19 Notify MD of need for surgical or manual debridement
	3.20 Following debridement apply a type of absorptive dressing • See procedure for application and changing of pressure ulcer dressing
STAGE FOUR:	3.21 Seek Skin Care Team evaluation of indication for use of specialty bed
	3.22 Institute interventions as used in previous stages as appropiate
	3.23 Follow pre-op orders if skin flap operation is planned
	3.24 Follow post-op orders after skin flap
4. EVALUATION:	4.1 Evaluate all high-risk patients: • On admission • With any change in skin integrity • With each dressing change
5. TEACHING/ INFORMATION	5.1 Instruct patient/significant other during hospital stay and at discharge on these principles: • Skin areas at greatest risk • Pressure relief/body mechanics • Cleansing skin/wound care • Dressing application • Nutritional maintenance • Importance of turning/activity schedule • Signs/symptoms of local/systemic infection
6. COMPLICATIONS: WORSENING ULCERATION	6.1 Notify Skin Care Team
FORMATION OF NEW ULCER	6.2 Notify Skin Care Team
INFECTION	6.3 Notify Skin Care Team if symptoms of systemic infection
	6.4 Obtain wound C&S • Refer to procedure
	6.5 Consult with infection control nurse • Refer to isolation procedure
7. DOCUMENTATION ASSESSMENT FORM	7.1 Indicate on body diagram location of redness or pressure ulcer on admission
	7.2 Describe ulcer by size, stage, depth, condition of wound base, presence of drainage, odor, signs and symptoms of infection, etc.
PROGRESS NOTES	7.3 Document and describe as above any pressure ulcers that develop
	7.4 Document and describe any complications that develop
	7.5 Instructions to family or patient
	7.6 Statement of progress toward healing with each dressing change
	7.7 Practice Guideline for Alteration in Skin Integrity implemented (include time and date)
ALTERATIONS IN SKIN INTEGRITY FLOW SHEET	7.8 Fill in required blanks on flow sheet

■ **FIGURE 7-4, cont'd.**

TYPE OF STANDARD

Clinical

PERSONNEL

RN

LPN (may perform labor observation and inspection and routine interventions 3.1.1-3.1.2)

COMPETENCIES

1. Perform vaginal examination
2. Insert IUPC
3. Interpret IUPC and fetal monitor patterns
4. Perform nipple stimulation
5. Place EFM
6. Perform Leopold maneuvers
7. Perform abdominal palpations of contractions

PATIENT OUTCOMES

1. Three contractions within a 10-minute window
2. External monitoring: firm contractions lasting 45-60 seconds
3. Internal monitoring; quality of contractions should be over 50 mm of pressure during contractions and 5-15 mm resting tone
4. Absence of complications/emergencies during labor

SUPPORTIVE DATA

Credentialed RN may insert IUPC

AREA OF RESPONSIBILITY	NURSING ORDERS
1. Assessment	
1.1 Maternal	1.1.1 Perform hands-on uterine assessment every hour and Leopold manevers as necessary
	1.1.2 Monitor uterine patterns continuously if internal monitor is in place
	1.1.3 Check bladder for distention every hour
	1.1.4 Perform vaginal examination as indicated by contractions and characteristics of labor progression
1.2 Fetal	1.2.1 Monitor FHT continuously by EFM
	1.2.2 Report to MD the following changes in FHT: a. increasing baseline b. decreased variability c. nonreassuring decelerations
	1.2.3 Observe fetal movement associated with 15×15 accelerations
	1.2.4 Report to MD decreasing accelerations or inability to elicit an acceleration with scalp stimulation
2. Planning	2. Collaborate with MD upon initiating protocol to determine individual modifications

■ FIGURE 7-5   Practice guidelines for patients with failure to progress.

AREA OF RESPONSIBILITY	NURSING ORDERS
3. Interventions	
3.1 Routine	3.1.1 Walk patient as tolerated
	3.1.2 Nipple stimulation according to procedure
	3.1.3 Insert intrauterine pressure catheter (IUPC) per MD order and procedure
	3.1.4 Place EFM as standard or IFM per MD order
	3.1.5 Begin Pitocin drip per MD order
	3.1.6 Increase infusion rate q 15 minutes to maximum of 20 milliunits
3.2 Complications/Emergencies	
3.2a Uterine rupture	a.1 Start IV infusion with NSS or LR if not already present
	a.2 Bolus with IV solution
	a.3 Obtain blood for type and cross match
	a.4 Start O_2/face mask at 10 L/minute
	a.5 Prep patient for C-section
3.2b Hyperstimulation of contraction patterns	b. In the presence of more than 5 contractions in a 10 minute window regardless of the quality of contractions
	1. Turn off Pitocin drip
	2. Place patient in left lateral position through 2 contractions, then right lateral position through 2 contractions
	3. If above ineffective, place patient in modified Trendelenburg with left lateral tilt
	4. Notify MD
3.2c Fetal distress	c.1 Place patient in left lateral position
	c.2 Turn off Pitocin drip
	c.3 Administer O_2/face mask at 10 L/minute
	c.4 Start fluid challenge with mainline IV solution
	c.5 Perform vaginal examination for presenting part and descent
	c.6 Manually elevate presenting part
	c.7 Notify MD stat
3.3 Patient information	3.3.1 Maintain left lateral position as much as possible
	3.3.2 Utilize breathing techniques during contractions
4. Outcome Evaluation	4. Evaluate progress toward outcomes q 15 minutes
5. Documentation	
5.1 Hollister Form	5.1.1 Chart timing, duration, quality of and FHT q 15 minutes
	5.1.2 Chart implementation of protocol
	5.1.3 Chart Pitocin administration and increases in drip rate
5.2 Patient Progress Record	5.2.1 Chart evaluative note qh

Authors: Marge Zerbe, RN
              Jacqueline Katz, MS, RN
References: John Smith, MD
Distribution: Labor and Delivery Department
Approval: 9/29/89
              Clinical Practice Council
Review: 9/29/90

■ FIGURE 7-5, cont'd.

into outcome indicators. For example, using the practice guidelines for the management of failure to progress in labor (Figure 7-5), any one or all of these four outcomes could be monitored:

$$\frac{\text{The number of patients with failure to progress}}{\text{achieving three contractions within a 10-minute period}}$$
$$\text{The total number of patients with failure to progress}$$

$$\frac{\text{The number of patients achieving firm, quality contractions}}{\text{lasting 45 to 60 seconds}}$$
$$\frac{\text{The total number of patients with failure to progress}}{\text{universe} = \text{externally monitored patients}}$$

$$\frac{\text{The number of patients with uterine contractions}}{\text{over 50 mm of pressure and 5 to 15 mm resting tone}}$$
$$\frac{\text{The total number of patients with failure to progress}}{\text{universe} = \text{internally monitored patients}}$$

$$\frac{\text{The number of patients experiencing complications}}{\text{or emergencies related to failure to progress}}$$
$$\text{The total number of patients with failure to progress}$$

Outcome indicators based on the alterations in skin integrity practice guidelines (Figure 7-4) might include:

$$\frac{\text{The number of incontinent (urine and stool) patients}}{\text{whose skin integrity declined during hospitalization}}$$
$$\frac{\text{The total number of incontinent patients}}{\text{(urine and stool)}}$$

$$\frac{\text{The number of patients 75 years of age or older with preexisting lesions}}{\text{whose lesions improved during hospitalization}}$$
$$\frac{\text{The total number of hospitalized patients 75 years of age or older}}{\text{with preexisting lesions}}$$

Various outcome indicators could be developed by combining specific aspects of the indications for implementing this practice guideline and the desired patient outcomes.

Process indicators could also be chosen from the nursing orders based on those interventions deemed essential to achievement of the stated outcomes.

Professional and administrative indicators are developed in much the same way as clinical indicators. For example, an important aspect of professional practice is the nursing process. The type or level of staff involved is the primary nurse and the primary associate. Related problems might include a lack of consistency in the use of nursing diagnosis terminology and poor documentation of evaluation of patient outcomes. A possible indicator might be:

$$\frac{\text{The number of primary nurses who use nursing diagnosis terminology}}{\text{The total number of primary nurses}}$$

Another indicator might be:

$$\frac{\text{The number of primary nurses who document evaluation of patient outcomes}}{\text{The total number of primary nurses}}$$

An important aspect of administrative practice might be budgeting. The type and level of staff involved might be nurse managers.

Problems related to this important aspect of service might include submission of incomplete budgets, late submission of budgets, and discrepancies between projected and actual budgets. Indicators might be written as:

$$\frac{\text{The number of incomplete budgets submitted}}{\text{The number of budgets submitted}}$$

and

$$\frac{\text{The number of budgets submitted by written deadline}}{\text{The total number of budgets submitted}}$$

and

$$\frac{\text{The number of budgets with negative discrepancies between actual and projected} > 10\%}{\text{The total number of budgets}}$$

The first two examples are process indicators, the third is an outcome indicator.

In designing indicators for a given aspect of care, practice, or governance, it is important to determine the true or potential problems that impede the pursuit of quality. These are the issues requiring the greatest attention in monitoring. Focusing on these issues will ensure that the monitoring and evaluation activities are relevant.

Developing indicators can be an overwhelming task. Where does one start? How does one decide what is an indicator? To assist in the design of indicators and to ensure that they are linked to written standards, we designed the indicator development form (see Figure 8-4). Based on the Joint Commission prototype Clinical Indicator Development Form, this form facilitates indicator development applicable to the important aspects of service defined in step 3.

Determining an indicator and setting its threshold are parts of the same process. This chapter focuses on indicator development. Setting thresholds is the focus of Chapter 8. Since the indicator development form includes both steps of the ten-step process, it is described in detail at the end of that chapter.

Indicators provide order within our lives. They keep us on track and provide clues that prod us to act both positively and negatively. Indicators in health care serve the same function. They are the "red flags" that indicate when quality falls below a predetermined acceptable level.

Good indicators are derived from well written standards. Without well written standards, it is impossible to design relevant indicators.

REFERENCES

1. Crosby PB: Quality is free, New York, 1979, New American Library.
2. Joint Commission on Accreditation of Healthcare Organizations: Characteristics of Clinical Indicators, Qual Rev Bulletin 15(11):330-339, 1989.
3. Joint Commission perspectives 10(1):6-7, 1990.
4. Joint Commission perspectives 10(6):1, 1990.
5. O'Leary D: The Joint Commission's Agenda for Change—stimulating continual improvement in the quality of care, Presented at AONE preconference, Baltimore, May 14, 1990.
6. O'Leary D: President's column, Joint Commission perspectives, pp 2, 3, July/August 1989.
7. Olivas G et al: Case management: a bottom line care delivery model, J Nurs Admin 19(11): 16-20, 1989.
8. Primer on Indicator Development and Application, Chicago, Joint Commission on Accreditation of Healthcare Organizations, 1991.
9. Treece E and Treece J: Elements of research in nursing, ed 3, St. Louis, 1982, The CV Mosby Co.

8

STEP 5:
ESTABLISHING THRESHOLDS
FOR EVALUATION

Quality is a matter of perception and,
like beauty, lies in the eyes of the beholder.
ELLIE GREEN

Torrential rain cascaded over John's shoulders from his ranger's hat. As he inched his way along the catwalk of the dam, he was grateful for the almost constant lightning that acted as backup to his flashlight.

At last he reached the gauges. Carefully he leaned over the edge of the dam to read the water level indicator. At midnight it had risen an inch above the yellow warning line and, according to policy, he had alerted the mayor to the possible need for an emergency evacuation of the town below.

At 1 AM, as the storm continued to rage, John again was peering at the gauges to see whether the water level had reached the red danger line. If so, he would initiate the evacuation plan adopted by the town council 6 months earlier. He hoped it would not be necessary. He knew how frightened his wife Mary would be if the evacuation alarm were sounded on such a stormy night.

In this story, John's thresholds for evaluation were clearly established: when the water level reached the yellow line the mayor was notified of the problem. If the rain had continued, causing the water level to rise to the red line, the town would be evacuated.

The threshold clearly delineated the acceptable level of safety or tolerance; exceeding that level would be John's signal to initiate immediate action. The yellow line served as a caution point. The red line served as the danger point—the point at which immediate action would be taken.

In other words, John relied upon established thresholds—the yellow and red lines—to provide the data necessary for the decision-making process.

■ DEFINITION OF THRESHOLDS

There are many thresholds in health care organizations. These thresholds are so common they often go unnoticed. For example, the blood pH threshold is 7.35 to 7.45. If a patient's pH deviates from this acceptable threshold, then a physician is notified at once. Insulin has a threshold relating to its shelf-life, which specifies the amount of time the solution is viable. In the coronary care department, thresholds for patients' heart rate and rhythm alarms are routinely set. In labor and delivery patients, fetal heart monitor alarm thresholds are also set. Such thresholds are used daily by staff members in all health care organizations in making decisions about patient care.

Obviously, the concept of thresholds is neither new nor mysterious, but rather, part of the daily work experience of all staff members. A new emphasis, however, has been accorded to thresholds in step 5 of the Joint Commission's ten-step process.

According to the Joint Commission, a threshold is "a level or point at which the results of data collection in monitoring and evaluation trigger intensive evaluation of a particular important aspect of care to determine whether an actual problem or opportunity for improvement exists."[1]

■ CHARACTERISTICS OF THRESHOLDS

A threshold is the border between compliance and noncompliance with written standards. Compliance is a positive factor. It signifies adherence or conformance to written standards. When staff are in compliance, they deliver patient care in accordance with the structure, process, outcome, and evaluation standards set by the organization. Compliance is composed of those controllable factors that affect quality outcomes. These might include the patient's understanding of the treatment plan, the staff's competence, or the availability of system resources. When all patient, staff, and system variables are controlled that can be, compliance is optimal. When patient, staff, and system variables are not fully controlled—i.e., they are not up to standard—compliance decreases and quality suffers.

Noncompliance is the lack of adherence or conformance to written standards. Noncompliance is a negative factor. When staff does not deliver services according to the structure process, outcome, and evaluation standards set by the organization, noncompliance exists. A portion of noncompliance is caused by patient, staff, and system variables that are less than optimal. When these variables are not fully controlled, noncompliance increases. A portion of noncompliance is also the result of chance or individual differences. This is the portion of noncompliance which is not controllable under any circumstances. For example, the patient's anatomy, the staff's intellectual capabilities, or the physical plant may be uncontrollable variables. The portion of noncompliance allowable in rate-based indicators is the portion that is not controllable.

As stated, the point that separates compliance from noncompliance is the threshold. Let us look at a clinical example.

The written standard states that patients' call bells will be answered within 3 minutes. In the specific department, it is determined that this standard can be adhered to 95% of the time. In other words, 95 out of 100 call bells will be answered within 3 minutes of being rung by a patient. This is a rate-based indicator and the compliance is 95%. The threshold measures compliance or how often something was done or achieved. Thus, if the rate of answering call bells within 3 minutes drops below 95%, further investigation of the variation would be required.

The same situation can be looked at from the opposite perspective, i.e., how many times call bells will not be answered within 3 minutes. This perspective focuses on noncompliance or how often something is not done or achieved. In this example, we would expect that no more than 5 out of 100 call bells would not be answered. The noncompliance is 5%. Should the number of call bells not answered exceed 5%, further investigation of the variation would be indicated.

Compliance and noncompliance are two sides of the same coin and the threshold is the dividing line. One hundred percent minus the percentage of noncompliance equals the percentage of compliance. Alternatively, one hundred percent minus the percentage of compliance equals the percentage of noncompliance.

The Joint Commission will accept either a threshold that specifies a level of compliance or one that specifies a level of noncompliance, provided that one type of threshold is used consistently throughout the division and is defined in writing.[4]

If adherence to standards (compliance) is being monitored, thresholds will be written that are high, i.e., closer to 100%. If, however, negative occurrences (noncompliance) are being monitored, thresholds will be written that are low, i.e., closer to 0%.

Thresholds are also dynamic. They change with continual improvement. Like performance, thresholds should improve over time. However, there comes a point in continual improvement when all the variables have been controlled that can be. There may always be some variables that cannot be controlled. When service is at its optimum level of quality, the emphasis is then placed on maintaining that level of quality while streamlining the process.

Thresholds also must be realistic. That is, they need to be feasible given the range of patient, staff, or system capabilities. Setting unachievable thresholds can quickly undermine quality improvement efforts. When establishing thresholds, keep in mind the uncontrollable factors that affect achievement. Many staff have difficulty accepting a threshold lower than 100% compliance or greater than 0% noncompliance. Except for sentinel events, such extremes may be noble, but are not realistic for most indicators.

To set absolute thresholds for every indicator being monitored is to program the system for failure. Staff become frustrated with the amount of review required since an inquiry is needed for all deviations from 100% compliance or 0% noncompliance. The system becomes administratively unmanageable because of the additional paperwork required; quality monitoring becomes a tedious exercise rather than the vital tool it was intended to be.

Lastly, thresholds are objective. They are the unbiased signs that mark the need for further investigation of an aspect of care/service. They are the benchmark against which current and future performance is and will be evaluated.

■ SETTING THRESHOLDS

There are two types of occurrences for which thresholds are set: sentinel events and rate-based events.

Thresholds for sentinel events are absolute. The threshold for compliance is 100% while the threshold for noncompliance is 0%. There is no tolerance for error. For example, all policies must always be adhered to without exception. There should be no tolerance for self-extubation, sponges left in the abdomen postoperatively, or administration of incompatible blood. Because the tolerance level is zero, each of these situations must be evaluated whenever it occurs. Immediate action must be taken to investigate the cause and to prevent recurrence.

On the other hand, the threshold for compliance in rate-based indicators is less than 100%, while the threshold for noncompliance exceeds 0%. Because the indicators being studied have been derived from the important aspects of care in the department, the compliance thresholds will, of course, be high. Noncompliance thresholds for these important aspects of care are set as close to zero as is feasible. Because these are critical aspects of care/service, most of the quality variables should be controlled, leaving only a small percentage of nonconformance because of uncontrollable factors.

■ ESTABLISHING A DESIRED THRESHOLD

Few organizations have developed national data bases upon which to base the selection of thresholds; however, the Joint Commission is working toward creating such a data base. It is their goal "to establish affordable mechanisms for the Joint Commission and health care organizations to support data collection, transmission, analysis and feedback." This set of activities will serve as a precursor to the development of an interactive data base through which trends in performance can be noted and individual organizations can compare their performance to that of others.[1]

Thresholds should never be set arbitrarily or they will have no basis in reality. Those who set thresholds arbitrarily frequently set a threshold that is unrealistic.

Making the transition to a statistically based monitoring program requires that thresholds be set that are statistically sound. In this method, a baseline threshold is defined as a starting point for the process of continual improvement. A retrospective analysis of a representative sample of the indicator population from the previous year is conducted to provide a baseline for the next year's threshold. The intensive retrospective analysis of past performance for the designated indicator on the basis of a large representative sample, increases the statistical significance of the baseline threshold. The results of this analysis serve as the baseline threshold.

For example, the indicator to be evaluated might be the effectiveness of diabetic patient teaching. It may be determined that the desired outcome of insulin administration instruction is the patient's ability to administer safely and correctly insulin at home within the first 48 hours after discharge. Thus, patients with a primary diagnosis of diabetes mellitus who returned to the emergency department (ED) within 48 hours of discharge with a diagnosis of insulin shock or ketoacidosis would indicate the inability of these patients to carry out the procedure correctly. These patients become the indicator population. An analysis of the previous year's ED admissions indicates admissions for 130 such patients. A random sample of 50 of these patients' charts is examined. Review of the charts demonstrates that in 10% of the cases, the patients either did not receive instruction in insulin administration or were unable to successfully prepare and administer the injection. Thus 10% becomes the baseline mean threshold for measuring noncompliance. The mean threshold for compliance is 90%.

This sort of retrospective analysis should be done before the start of any monitoring cycle and should also be included as part of the annual summary report on each indicator so that the following year's threshold can be set using the previous year's data.

This method quickly provides a historical overview of performance and a baseline for the following year's threshold. The authors recognize that for high-volume indicators, the sample numbers required to obtain statistical significance may appear prohibitive when resources such as time and staff are constrained. However, the move to a statistically based quality monitoring program cannot occur without the commitment of the resources necessary to provide accurate baseline data upon which to monitor current practice and plan for future improvement.

Once obtained, the mean baseline threshold is then compared to the ideal threshold that has been established. The discrepancy is calculated by subtracting the baseline from the ideal. For example, a panel of experts decides that 95% of the patients receiving instruction regarding insulin administration should be able to carry out the procedure correctly within 48 hours of their discharge from the hospital. Subtracting

90% (last year's performance) from 95% yields a discrepancy of 5%. There is a difference of 5% between the baseline threshold, i.e., the present threshold, and the ideal threshold, the desired threshold. If the discrepancy is greater than 10% and if it is also the opinion of the experts that this discrepancy is controllable—i.e., performance can be improved by correcting patient, staff, or system variables—then a concurrent monitoring study should be done to confirm that actual practice is at the baseline threshold. If the discrepancy is less than 10%, the ideal threshold becomes the desired threshold for the initial monitoring study.

To determine how much improvement must be achieved in each monitoring study, the discrepancy between actual and ideal performance is divided by the number of monitoring studies proposed for the upcoming year minus 1, to determine the incremental improvement necessary for the period between two sequential monitoring studies.

■ THRESHOLD PARAMETERS VERSUS ABSOLUTE THRESHOLDS

There is variability in everything. For example, the likelihood that an expert marksman will hit the bull's-eye each time is determined by the individual's proficiency. However, the likelihood that the exact same hole in the bull's-eye will be hit each time is less assured. There is normal variance in performance. This applies to quality monitoring also.

Suppose we have set a threshold for compliance of 97%. Theoretically, this means that if we do not achieve that precise threshold each time we monitor, additional analysis is necessary. The likelihood of hitting the 97% mark precisely in each of the four monitoring studies is low, just as the likelihood that the marksman will hit the same bullet hole each time is low. We aim to hit the bull's-eye, not necessarily the same bullet hole. As long as the bull's-eye is hit each time, the marksman is a winner. The bull's-eye is an area, not a pinpoint. It would be much more difficult for a marksman, no matter how skilled, to repetitively hit a bull's-eye the size of the bullet.

We want to provide staff with an *area* of quality success to aim for, not a pinpoint target. Setting threshold parameters provides the limits within which it can safely be said that quality exists. It is similar to stating that a normal patient blood pressure reading is 120/80. While 120/80 is recognized as the norm, some variation is expected. Even if an initial reading is 120/80, at a later time it may be 115/85. The medical profession has established parameters for blood pressure which are reasonable and safe. A blood pressure reading between 100/60 and 140/90 is generally considered acceptable, but beyond that range, the physician may decide to take action.

Why? Because historically, positive patient outcomes are associated with blood pressures within the acceptable range while negative outcomes are reported when the blood pressure falls outside those parameters. In other words, there are acceptable threshold parameters for blood pressure readings.

Setting thresholds as absolutes, except for sentinel events, places an undue burden on practitioners to "hit the mark" every time. Furthermore, it promotes unproductive and undesirable reactions: any time staff fails to "hit the mark" they feel that they are not fully competent. Staff members can become discouraged with the process, which may hinder the entire monitoring program. In their frustration over lack of achievement, their morale may suffer. Staff does not want to participate in activities that constantly make them feel inadequate. They may be reluctant to participate in future monitoring activities or recalcitrant with regard to quality improvement efforts. Worse yet, they may choose to hide (or not report) monitoring results that are less than perfect. Therefore, it is far better to set threshold parameters than absolute

COL 1	COL 2	COL 3	COL 4
MONTHS	TOTAL MEDICATION ERRORS x_i	DEVIATIONS $x_i - \bar{x}$	SQUARE OF DEVIATIONS $(x_i - \bar{x})^2$
JAN	10	0	0
FEB	12	2	4
MAR	11	1	1
APR	8	−2	4
MAY	11	1	1
JUN	9	−1	1
JUL	7	−3	9
AUG	10	0	0
SEP	12	2	4
OCT	10	0	0
NOV	13	3	9
DEC	7	−3	9
	TOTAL: **120**		TOTAL: **42**

- $\bar{x} = \dfrac{\Sigma x_i}{N} = \dfrac{120}{12} = 10$

- $\sigma = \sqrt{\dfrac{\Sigma(x_i - \bar{x})^2}{N}} = \sqrt{\dfrac{42}{12}} = \sqrt{3.5} = \pm 1.9$

- Threshold parameters
    Upper limit: $\bar{x} + \sigma = 10 + 1.9 = 11.9$
    Lower limit: $\bar{x} - \sigma = 10 - 1.9 = 8.1$

(x_i = individual score; $\bar{x}$ = mean (or average) of scores; N = number of scores; σ = standard deviation)

1. Enter the number of medication errors reported each month in column 2.
2. Total the entries in column 2 to determine the annual total of the medication errors reported.
3. Divide the total calculated in step 2 by the number of months for which medication error date is available.
   Note: This quotient is $\bar{x}$, the mean, or average number of reported medication errors per month.
4. Subtract the calculated average ($\bar{x}$) from each reported number of monthly medication errors, and enter the deviations ($x_i - \bar{x}$) in column 3.
   Note: Values may be positive, negative, or zero.
5. Multiply each calculated deviation by itself, and enter the resultant products in column 4.
   Note: All values will be positive, or zero.
6. Add the products in column 4. To determine the sum of squared deviations [$\Sigma(x_i - \bar{x})^2$]
7. Divide the sum calculated in step 6 by the number of months for which medication error data is available.
8. Calculate the square root of the quotient determined in step 7.
   Note: This calculation yields σ, the standard deviation of the data entered in column 2.
9. Calculate:
   - the upper limit of the threshold parameters, $\bar{x} + \sigma$, by adding the calculated standard deviation (σ, see step 8) to the calculated average ($\bar{x}$, step 3), and
   - the lower limit of the threshold parameters, $\bar{x} - \sigma$, by subtracting the calculated standard deviation (σ, see step 8) from the calculated average ($\bar{x}$, step 3).

■ **FIGURE 8-1**   Nine-step procedure for calculating a standard deviation and confidence interval.

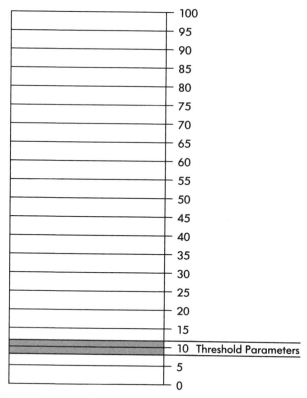

■ FIGURE 8-2   Medication error threshold parameters 8.1 to 11.9.

thresholds. Threshold parameters define the upper and lower limits of acceptance for the results of a monitoring study.

Thresholds for evaluation may be statistically determined control limits, specification limits, trends, or patterns. They are mechanisms used to determine when processes or outcomes of care must be further evaluated. Thresholds help determine when unexpected or possibly undesirable occurrences must be evaluated (e.g. in QI terms, "the process is out of control"). However, evaluation may (and in QI often does) occur even when thresholds are not crossed. In such circumstances, the evaluation process uses the indicator data to better understand current performance and its causes in order to develop strategies for future improvement.[2]

Statistically correct parameters are really upper and lower control limits set above and below a desired mean. Calculating statistically accurate parameters requires a retrospective analysis of the indicator and the calculation of its standard deviation. This will provide the most accurate calculation of the threshold parameters and allow much more reliable prediction of the results of future monitoring studies. The authors again acknowledge that this type of analysis may require the commitment of resources that may not be available at the department level. This type of statistical analysis as a precursor to monitoring may fall within the realm of the quality management council. Many individual organizations look to national organizations and the development of national data bases as an alternative to this analysis; however, these alternatives will not provide the same individualized data as an internal baseline.

Figure 8-1 shows a nine-step procedure for manually calculating a standard deviation and threshold parameters. In the example shown in Figure 8-1, the threshold interval limits or threshold parameters are 8.1 to 11.9. Figure 8-2 is a schematic diagram of these parameters. Automated calculation of standard deviation coupled with

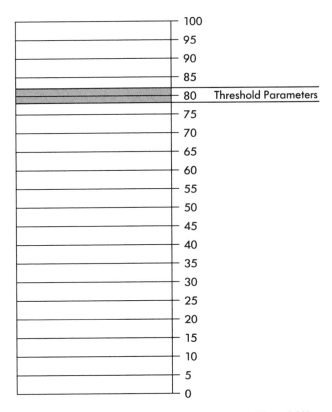

■ **FIGURE 8-3**   **Threshold parameters: 78% to 82%.**

automated data collection can streamline the process of setting statistically meaningful thresholds and threshold parameters.

A less desirable and less accurate way to set threshold parameters is to review the sample data from the baseline threshold and determine a range that is equidistant from the threshold. For example, if the baseline threshold is 80%, plus or minus 2% may be regarded as an acceptable range. Thus the threshold parameters would become 78 to 82%, as is depicted in Figure 8-3. If the results of a monitoring study fall within that range, they are judged to be successful and quality is maintained for that indicator. Consensus-based threshold parameters should allow for variation in performance that is caused by chance but should not be so wide as to be nondiscriminating. That is, they should allow for chance occurrences but should not allow for variation based on controllable patient, staff, or system variables. This method is not precise and should be used only during an initial monitoring cycle (1 year). The data provided during this monitoring cycle will afford the necessary information for performing the statistical analysis described earlier. The authors recommend that as a part of the annual summary report on each indicator, a formal statistical analysis of standard deviation be done so that the next year's threshold and threshold parameters can be set with confidence.

■ THE INDICATOR DEVELOPMENT FORM

In Chapter 7 we discussed the process of developing indicators and data elements. In this chapter we have considered setting thresholds and threshold parame-

Text continues on p. 118.

Developed by: _____ Date: _____

1. Important Aspect of Care, Practice, Governance: _____

Indicator Populations	Definitions of Terms and Tools:
1.	
2.	
3.	

Patient Variables

1. _____
2. _____
3. _____

Staff Variables

1. _____
2. _____
3. _____

System Variables

1. _____
2. _____
3. _____

Indicator	Threshold Parameters	Related Standards	Data Elements	Data Sources
A. Structure ☐ Process ☐ Outcome ☐		1. 2. 3.	1. 2. 3.	1. 2. 3.
B. Structure ☐ Process ☐ Outcome ☐		1. 2. 3.	1. 2. 3.	1. 2. 3.
C. Structure ☐ Process ☐ Outcome ☐		1. 2. 3.	1. 2. 3.	1. 2. 3.

■ FIGURE 8-4   Indicator development form. (© 1991 Jackie Katz and Ellie Green. Reprinted with permission.)

1. Important Aspect of (Care) Practice, Governance: Developed by: _Oncology Unit QMC_   Date: _12·17·9-_

Pain Management

Indicator Populations	Definitions of Terms and Tools:
1. Ca, breast (Drgs: 274, 275)	1. McGill Pain Scale [2] (see attached)
	2. Acute Pain: intense and of short duration (< 6 mos.)
2. Ca, lung (Drg: 282)	3. Chronic pain: longer duration (> 6 mos.), continuous or intermittent, can be intense
3. Ca, Colon (Drgs: 172, 173)	4. PCAU: Patient Controlled Analgesia Unit
	5. Terminal: Predicted life expectancy < 3 months

Patient Variables
1. Ability or will to participate in pain control i.e. the use of PCAU
2. Pain tolerance (affected by age, sex, duration of pain, severity of illness)
3. Fear and Anxiety level

Staff Variables
1. Personal frame of reference related to pain
2. Knowledge of pain theory and management
3. _____

System Variables
1. # of credentialed (pain) nurses/shift
2. # of PCAUs available
3. _____

Indicator	Threshold Parameters	Related Standards	Data Elements	Data Sources
A. Structure ☐ Process ☐ Outcome ☐ Numerator: # of Terminal Ca Patients using PCAU who express level 0-1 on McGill Pain Scale Denominator: Total # of Terminal Ca Patients	85-95%	1. Practice Guideline for Management of Acute Pain 2. PCAU Procedure 3.	1. Terminal Ca 2. PCAU in use 3. RN's comfort level	1. Patients' progress record 2. observation 3. Patient interview, Patients' progress record
B. Structure ☐ Process ☐ Outcome ☐ Numerator: # of oncology RNs certified in pain control management Denominator: Total # of oncology RNs	90-100%	1. Core Curriculum for Pain management 2. 3.	1. Score ≥ 90% on credentialing exam 2. 3.	1. exam scores 2. 3.
C. Structure ☐ Process ☐ Outcome ☐ Numerator: # of PCAUs in use on Terminal Ca Patients Denominator: Total # of Terminal Ca Patients able to participate in PCAU	90-100%	1. Goal related to resource availability on PCAU 2. 3.	1. # Terminal Ca Patient 2. PCAUs available 3. # of Terminal Ca Patients	1. Observation 2. Unit Inventory 3. Census

■ FIGURE 8-5 Completed indicator development form. (© 1991 Jackie Katz and Ellie Green. Reprinted with permission.)

ters. Since these processes are interdependent, the authors designed an indicator development form that encompasses both processes. The form is based on The Joint Commission's suggested indicator development form format. The form, depicted in Figure 8-4, integrates written standards as a basis for indicator development, the process of developing indicators, and threshold development.

The following are directions for completing the form.

Step 1: Important Aspects of Care, Practice, or Governance. After choosing an important aspect of care, practice, or governance from the priority list, circle the appropriate word and write the topic in the blank provided. List the individual or group who developed the indicator and the date.

Step 2: Indicator Populations. List no more than three populations for whom this important aspect is critical. Target populations for monitoring will be chosen from this list.

Step 3: Definition of Terms and Tools. List any terms or tools associated with the important aspect. Define any terms that may have multiple interpretations, including acronyms and abbreviations or terms that have a specific meaning particular to a department or division. Attach a copy of any tools related to the important aspect (e.g., the Norton scale for pressure ulcer staging) or a classification tool for severity of medication errors. Uniform definitions ensure uniform understanding and greater accuracy and reliability in data collection.

Step 4: Patient Variables (related to the important aspect being studied). Identify up to three variables related to the patient that may have a direct impact on achievement of quality within the important aspect under investigation. These can be controllable or uncontrollable factors and might include age, sex, comorbidity, educational level, and so on.

Step 5: Staff Variables (related to important aspect being studied). Identify up to three variables related to the staff that may have a direct impact on the achievement of quality within the important aspect under investigation. These can be controllable or uncontrollable factors and might include years of experience, credentials, academic preparation, and so on.

Step 6: System Variables (related to important aspect being studied). Identify up to three variables related to the system that may have a direct impact on the achievement of quality within the important aspect under investigation. These can be controllable or uncontrollable factors and might include staffing, work shift differences, budget constraints, equipment availability, and so on.

Step 7: Indicators. Three boxes labelled A, B, and C provide space for the development of indicators related to the important aspect of care, practice, or governance identified in step 1. Use the information in steps 2 through 6 to assist in the development of specific indicators. Enter one indicator per box. Remember to write each indicator as a ratio. Check the appropriate small box indicating that the indicator is structure, process, or outcome.

Step 8: Threshold Parameters. Enter the threshold parameters that have been set for each indicator.

Step 9: Standards Identification. List the structure, process, or outcome standards that are related to the indicator to be studied as identified in step 1.

Step 10: Data Elements. List up to three data elements that are specific to this indicator. These are chosen directly from the indicator itself.

Step 11: Data Sources. List the sources for retrieval of information for each data
element listed in step 10. Sources can be documentation, observation, interview, and the like.

Figure 8-5 shows a completed form, using the example of pain management.

Developing process or outcome indicators for important aspects of care, practice,
or governance focuses the monitoring activities on the three domains that control
quality. Using this method to develop indicators and threshold parameters may be a
dramatic departure from the traditional approach to quality assurance. This method,
however, fosters a standards-based approach to the development of quality indicators
and a statistical approach to setting the monitoring parameters. The data yielded by
these processes will ultimately more accurately and reliably represent the level of
quality within the division of nursing.

Once the indicator development form has been completed, the process of planning for data collection can begin.

REFERENCES

1. Agenda for Change kit, Chicago, 1990, Joint
   Commission on Accreditation of Healthcare
   Organizations.
2. Hospitals use M & E to improve quality, Joint
   Commission Perspectives 11(2):1, March/April
   1991.
3. Long B and Phipps W: Medical-surgical nursing, ed 2, St. Louis, 1989, The CV Mosby Co.
4. Personal communication: Carol Patterson, Director of Standards Interpretation, Joint Commission on Accreditation of Healthcare Organizations, 1988.

9

STEP 6:
COLLECTING AND ORGANIZING DATA

In God we trust. All others must use data.
W. EDWARDS DEMING

Well here I am, flat on my back literally and in other ways, right ankle resting on three pillows. Gravity is vital to treatment. . . .

Dr. Sch . . . ordered from the drug store (in the hospital) a paste for the itch that had set in Minneapolis. The drug store was out of one of the ingredients: must order it from the whole-saler, and can not make it up til Monday. I need it tonight. On prodding from Dr. Sch . . . the drug store sent someone out to another drug store to fetch the missing ingredient. The paste came up that evening.

Unbelievable: the same scenario took place some days later.

I wonder why is a registered nurse making beds? It seems to me that making beds is not good use of her time. Her education and skills could be put to better use, so it seems to me.

The chair in this room is huge, would seat two people, takes up an exorbitant amount of space, heavy to move. . . . The coat hangers here are that maddening kind, found in most hotels. . . .

My nurse of the moment put on a hot towel this afternoon. "I'll be back in twenty minutes, and if I don't come, please ring." Sixty-five minutes later I pressed the button. A helper came in; explained to me that this was not her kind of job, so she canceled the light for the nurse, and went off. Thirty minutes later I rang again for the nurse. The same helper came and observed again that the job was not her line of duty, so again she canceled the light and went off. The solution was simple, for me, merely discard the towel and insulation myself with the rules or against the rules. The same event recurred another day.

What is the moral of all this? What have we learned? One answer: the superintendent of the hospital needs to learn something about supervision. Only he can make the changes in procedure and responsibility that are required.

Talks between physicians and nurses, even with the head nurse, accomplish nothing. The same problems that I have noted will continue. A physician cannot change the system. A head nurse cannot change the system. Meanwhile, who would know? To work harder will not solve the problem. The nurses couldn't work any harder.[4]

Dr. Deming describes his hospitalization in graphic detail. He describes a scene that is familiar to many busy nurses. It is the sort of ordinary event that rarely becomes part of a monitoring and evaluation study. Why? Because most studies directed to-ward a patient's treatment ask the question, "was the treatment given?" and, in this case, the treatment was given. But the treatment was, to Dr. Deming, very unsatisfactory even though it may have been beneficial medically. So, how do we collect data on the many issues that irritate patients and frustrate nurses in a health care organization?

How do we change data collection from the traditional approach in which a staff member's completion of tasks is checked off a list to a more realistic approach in which meaningful data will be gathered about patient outcomes and reactions to treatment?

First, it is necessary to understand that the approach used depends on what sort of quality is to be improved. The two major forms of "quality" consist of:

1. Quality in the sense of "those product features which meet the needs of customers and thereby provide product satisfaction."[1] In short, patient satisfaction with our care and service.
2. "Quality in the sense of freedom from deficiencies."[1]

In health care, both of these two major forms of quality must be consistently measured and improved. The two forms cannot be separated. Then the new quality era arrives—and many health care professionals are struggling to hasten its arrival—data will be used to make a difference in patient care, professional practice, and governance! These data will provide information about the care and service delivered by health care organizations as well as the defects that occur.

Data collection is the backbone of a quality management program. Without accurate data, there cannot be accurate analysis or solutions.

"In God we trust. All others must use data." Mary Walton explains this Deming credo for improvement in *The Deming Management Method*. She states, "Critical to the Deming method is the need to base decisions as much as possible on accurate and timely data, not on wishes, hunches or 'experience.'"[3] The bumper sticker that proclaims "Accountants Do It with Data," while amusing, is not far off the mark. We quality management professionals would be wise to follow the credo of Deming and the accountants. We should make sure that we "do" all of our analyses and draw all our conclusions "with data."

A training manual for Komatsu Ltd., a Japanese competitor of Caterpillar Tractor Company, puts it this way: "The first step in quality is to judge and act on the basis of facts. Views not backed by data are more likely to include personal opinions, exaggeration and mistaken impressions."[3] If accurate data are of paramount importance in manufacturing tractors, consider how much more important they are in guiding health care professionals in making decisions about patient care, professional practice, and governance!

Unfortunately, much confusion surrounds data collection in today's health care organizations. The art of accurate data collection using simple statistics is new to many quality management professionals. When faced with the task of data collection, many professionals express concerns about basic concepts. Many ask questions such as:

- What are the goals of data collection?
- Who should collect data?
- In which domain?
- About what?
- For what purpose?
- What are the sources of data?
- What tools are used?

All of these questions need to be answered before data collection begins. Once these questions are addressed, data collection becomes a meaningful tool in the organization's decision-making process. When sound decisions are made, plans are carried out correctly the first time. Quality management professionals can make accurate decisions about conserving or expending resources when those decisions are rooted in accurate data.

■ THE GOALS OF DATA COLLECTION

Because accurate data collection is the cornerstone of quality management, data collection plays a vital role in the quality management process. The first goal of data collection is to establish a system to ensure accuracy of information on which to base future decisions. A poor decision made as the result of inaccurate data can result in harm to a patient, misspent funds, wasted time, improper utilization of personnel, inadequate or surplus purchases of equipment, the creation of inappropriate standards, and so on. Resources are precious in today's health care environment and a poor decision based on inaccurate data can be extremely costly to an organization.

The second goal of data collection is to avoid all punitive measures associated with the results of collected data. When workers feel that their jobs are threatened by the results of the data that they have collected, they may simply hide the data. This does not mean that they are "bad" employees. It simply means that they are employees who desperately depend on their income. If they feel that their job security is jeopardized by accurately reporting data, they may pursue a safe course and maintain the status quo. Dr. Deming says, "In the perception of most employees preserving the status quo is the only safe course."[3] The quality assurance professional should create an environment of nonpunitive, safe data reporting. Employees will cooperate with collecting and reporting data when they feel secure and unafraid of retaliation and negative consequences.

The third goal of data collection is to pinpoint the domain—clinical, professional, or administrative—that is in need of improvement. Once an important aspect of care or service is selected, monitoring focuses on all three domains. For example, the indicators chosen in Chapter 8 concern pain management of the oncology patient. Each of the indicators surrounding this important aspect of care deal with a specific domain. On the indicator development form shown in Figure 8-5, the indicator labelled *A* deals with the clinical domain, the indicator labelled *B* deals with the professional domain, and the indicator labelled *C* deals with the administrative domain. By using this trifocus approach, a picture emerges of pain control for terminal oncology patients. Now problems can be identified easily and solved in the appropriate domain.

The fourth goal of data collection is to identify actions or reasons that precipitated a sentinel event. Insofar as possible, sentinel events must not be permitted to occur. They are unusual occurrences and are generally associated with negative or adverse consequences to the patient, the staff, or the organization. The quality management council must investigate every sentinel event, examining all three domains to analyze the cause and effect of the occurrence.

The fifth goal of data collection is to establish the degree to which improvement has occurred after implementation of an action plan. Data collection is a futile exercise unless the information is used to create improvement in the care, practice, or governance of the organization. Data must be collected following the initiation of every action plan to either confirm or deny expected results.

The sixth goal is to collect data at regular intervals on all important aspects of care to demonstrate sustained improvement. This requires that data be used to track and discern trends in results over a period of time. The threshold parameter form (see Figure 10-4) is used for that purpose.

■ WHO SHOULD COLLECT DATA?

Data collection must be planned, organized, ongoing, and systematic. Achieving this requires organization as well as delegation of accountability and responsibility. The job is too big for one person to assume the responsibility for either organization-wide or department-based data collection. Therefore, quality management councils (QMC) are implemented throughout the division as well as in each department.

It is far more practical to place the responsibility and accountability for data collection with councils. The division of nursing QMC functions as the central quality resource center. This central council determines and delegates appropriate generic data collection to each of the department-based QMCs. Department-based QMCs, in turn, delegate this generic monitoring and data collection to their trained QMC staff members.

In addition to the generic division-wide activity, department-specific monitoring and evaluation are also continuous. But they are not independent of the division QMC. The division of nursing QMC functions as the central clearinghouse for *all* quality studies. Each department-based QMC regularly reports to the division QMC so that "the right hand knows what the left hand is doing."

Here is how it works: the division of nursing QMC develops from the important aspects of care and service the generic division-wide indicators to be monitored and prepares the data collection forms that accompany the indicators. These prepared data collection forms are then distributed to the department-based QMCs for data collection by their trained staff members. These department-based QMC staff members usually have attended an inservice program on the quality management data collection process and have been certified by the education department as data collectors. Once the generic data have been collected and analyzed the staff members return the results to the QMC for review and trend forecasting.

The department-based QMC members carry on a similar program of monitoring and evaluation in which they monitor the important aspects of care and service specific to their area. For example, the obstetrical department monitors fetal heart tones and epidural anesthesia, the coronary care department monitors the outcomes of intra-aortic balloon pump therapy, etc. However, all of their data will be passed on to the division-wide QMC at regular intervals.

In other words, each QMC—both division-wide and department-based—functions as a hub of quality activities. This hub, around which all quality management revolves, is necessary to achieve quality improvement within the organization because it provides a planned, systematic approach that does not depend on one person. Rather, councils composed of trained professionals plan, organize, direct, evaluate, and make decisions on where improvements are necessary within the division and within each department.

Neither division-wide quality, nor department-based quality can occur unless there is a governing *body* empowered with responsibility and accountability for quality. Quality is not analogous to a solo performance but rather to that of a symphony orchestra. When the quality activities of all departments are orchestrated with the division-wide QMC, there is a beauty of coordination that is exciting, fun, and inspiring to staff members.

This orchestration of efforts prevents duplication and waste of resources and provides structure for the improvement process. In order for the improvement process to occur, there must be a regular flow of consistent data. These data are then used to track and discern trends in results over a period of time. Improvement may then be made with solid, provable data instead of hunches, guesses, or opinions.

■ DATA SHOULD BE COLLECTED IN EACH DOMAIN

It is important that each important aspect of care/service have a trifocus. Indicators should be developed in the clinical, professional, and administrative domains. By developing an indicator for each of the domains—clinical, professional, and administrative—and collecting pertinent demographic data relating to the indicators, a complete picture emerges, and problems can be pinpointed or improvements made in the appropriate domain.

■ APPROPRIATE SUBJECTS FOR DATA COLLECTION

Not every aspect of care/service within a health care organization qualifies as a subject for monitoring. Since resources are scarce, monitoring should center around those important aspects of care and service that are high risk, high volume, problem prone, and high cost. Typically those subjects that are process related, that is, tasks that nurses routinely perform, are not good subjects for monitoring. It is not that the tasks are unimportant. Every nurse knows the importance of starting an IV, inserting a Foley catheter, changing a dressing, and suctioning a patient on a ventilator whose pressure alarm is sounding. Tasks are important, but whether or not a task was performed correctly will be manifested in patient outcomes. Therefore, patient outcomes will be the initial barometer of how well tasks were performed. For example, if the staff members are not inserting Foley catheters, changing dressings, or starting IVs using sterile technique it will quickly become apparent in an increase in urinary tract, surgical wound, and IV site infections. Patients who are not promptly suctioned while on the ventilator will hear the relentless alarm sounding until the "task" is performed properly. Therefore, it is the presence or absence of infections, the pressure build-up on the ventilator, and so on that should be monitored initially, not the tasks involved in the individual procedures. If there is an increased infection rate or if patients are consistently in distress while on the ventilator, an action plan should be developed to solve the problem. The action plan might include a refresher on sterile technique, an inservice presentation on ventilator care, and the like. Once the action plan has concluded, a new monitoring study of the infection rate and outcomes of ventilator care will validate the effectiveness of the action plan.

Just as data are collected about patient outcomes in the clinical domain, data on staff outcomes are collected in the professional domain, and data on system outcomes are collected in the administrative domain. In other words, outcomes are written in all three domains—clinical, professional, and administrative—and this trifocus should be used for all data collection.

An example of a clinical outcome for the procedure to insert a Foley catheter includes "the bladder will be drained." Examples of professional practice outcomes are found in every clinical procedure and in every practice guideline. For example, the procedure for inserting a Foley catheter might have the professional outcome: "Bladder catheterization accomplished maintaining sterility." If the nurse inserts the device using sterile technique it should be a relatively risk-free procedure to the patient. Staff outcomes may also be located in a practice guideline. For example, a staff outcome in the practice guideline for management of the patient with violent behavior might read: "absence of staff physical injury during patient's length of stay."

To complete the trifocus, data also should be collected about issues of governance in the administrative domain. System outcomes also may be found in procedures and practice guidelines. For example, in the procedure for applying restraints the system outcome might read: "the security restraint bag will be stocked and available on the crash cart rack at all times."

Appropriate subjects for data collection fall into all three domains. Organizations should not limit data collection to patient care or staff practices but also should include the domain of governance. In other words, data collection must include a broader focus than just the clinical aspects of patient care if it is to have an impact on continual improvement within the organization. This broader focus serves as a mandate to monitor critical aspects of care, practice, or governance that have a direct impact on the quality of patient care provided.

■ PURPOSE OF DATA COLLECTION

There are four important reasons to collect data. The first is to validate that things are happening the way the division of nursing plans for them to happen. Once a division of nursing creates a standards-based system, it will then monitor the standards to ensure that they are being adhered to by the staff members. This monitoring will produce data that will confirm or deny the efficacy of the standards.

The second reason for data collection is to provide a basis for change or improvement in the care, practice, or governance of the organization. Positive change or improvement is neither happenstance nor instantaneous. The Ford Motor Company did not go from producing the Model T to manufacturing the Taurus instantly or by chance! Without continuous research, data collection, and development, and without action on the data, the automobile industry might still be using a crank to start its engines. Health care also must continue to change, develop, and improve. Accurate data will lay the foundation for necessary change and continual improvement.

The third reason to collect data is to provide a rationale for increasing or decreasing resources, or maintaining the same level of resources within the organization. Health care organizations lack resources to hire, fire, purchase, plan, or govern based on a "hunch." Sound data collection can prevent the carrying out of inappropriate, costly "hunches." Accurate data ensure that the organization makes decisions based on factual information grounded in the realities of current practice.

A fourth reason to collect data is to provide a basis for the development of reliable thresholds for evaluation to be used in tracking and trending of care, practice, and governance of the organization. Without an historic data base, gathered over a period of months to years, threshold parameters are, at best, guesses. Thresholds will never be reliable until sound scientific and statistical methods are employed in their development. Accurate data are needed for thresholds to evolve into meaningful statistics that are beneficial to organizations.

■ SOURCES OF DATA WITHIN THE ORGANIZATION

Data come from three types of sources, which reflect the three domains of nursing: the consumer of the service, the deliverer of the service, and the management of the service. Some examples of consumer sources include the patient who receives the service, the family and significant others, and the community. Some examples of professional sources, or deliverers of service, include nursing staff members, physicians, and ancillary personnel. Management sources include nursing and hospital-wide administrators, and human resources managers.

All three data sources should be considered when designing the quality manage-

---

KATZ-GREEN GUIDELINES FOR MONITORING

TYPE OF STUDY	SAMPLE SIZE
Routine review	5% or 20 (whichever is greater)
Query review	10% or 40 (whichever is greater)
Intensive review	15% or 60 (whichever is greater)
Sentinel event	100% (every event)

---

ment program. Limiting data collection to one source will narrow the scope of the collection process and restrict its usefulness. Similarly, utilizing only one type of collection tool will limit the scope and narrow the focus of the collection process. Many different tools should be used.

■ HOW MUCH DATA SHOULD BE COLLECTED?

The volume of data to be collected will vary depending on the type of study being undertaken. As part of THE BLUEPRINT, the authors established the guidelines that appear in the box above to assist in determining appropriate sample sizes. Using these guidelines or developing similar guidelines of its own will help an organization establish some fundamental operating rules for monitoring. As would be expected, a query review requires a larger sample than a routine review, and a sentinel event necessitates investigation of every incident.

We recommend a sample size of 5% or 20, whichever is the larger for a routine review. The study may involve 20 charts, patients, nurses, doctors, and so on, depending on its focus.

A query review occurs when data demonstrate a variance outside the established threshold parameters that cannot readily be explained or justified. For a query review, we recommend a sample size of 10% or 40, whichever is greater. The study may involve 40 charts, patients, nurses, doctors, procedures, and so on, depending on its focus.

An intensive review is conducted when unusual occurrences or trends within the organization demonstrate a negative impact on patient outcomes. We recommend that intensive reviews use a sample size of 15% or 60, whichever is greater. The study may involve 60 charts, patients, nurses, doctors, procedures, and so on, depending on its focus.

The sentinel event review is conducted when adverse happenings extend a patient's length of stay in the facility, compromise a patient's quality of life, or cause death. Examples include exsanguination, airway obstruction, electrical hazards, medication errors resulting in death, administering the wrong blood type to a patient, and the like. Sentinel events require 100% compliance and monitoring every event.

■ TOOLS USED IN DATA COLLECTION

Seven different types of tools are typically used to collect data. They are:

- Data collection forms
- Forms for management rounds

- End-of-shift reports
- Suggestion boxes
- Satisfaction surveys
- Hot lines
- Focus groups

Data Collection Forms

Essential to any good quality management program is a data collection tool that is simple to understand, contains necessary data when completed, and is flexible enough to be used throughout the organization. THE BLUEPRINT contains a data collection form that has been widely tested in health care facilities and has met the criteria of understandability, pertinence, and flexibility (Figure 9-1). It has been designed to be used in conjunction with the indicator development form (see Figure 8-4). The indicator development form is always completed first, then the data collection form is filled in. Together, these forms provide a comprehensive yet easy-to-use data collection format for the quality professional. An explanation of how the data collection form is used follows. The numbers in the explanation correspond to the sections identified by number in Figure 9-1.

1. Fill in the date when data collection begins.
2. Fill in the date when the study ends.
3. Enter the name of the department in which the study is being conducted.
4. Enter a study number. Assigning study numbers permits easy comparison of data on graphic displays.
5. Identify the name of the person(s) collecting the data.
6. Enter the important aspect of care, service, or governance about which data are to be collected. Note that this will also have been designated on the indicator development form.
7. Check the appropriate box or boxes that describe whether the important aspect of care, service, or governance is high volume, high risk, problem prone, or high cost.
8. Indicate the sample size. Entering the sample size helps provide a complete picture of the study. For example: 20 of 250 patient charts; 20 of 42 ventilator patients; 20 of 57 staff members.
9. List any exceptions. Exceptions are those factors that would prevent the data elements from being evaluated. For example, if patients' verbal responses to pain management were the focus of a study and the sample size included every patient, then the comatose patient would be an exception.
10. The "Remarks" section is provided for the evaluator to record any pertinent information about the study that has no designated place on the form.
11. Identification numbers for up to 20 items in a sample are listed across the top of the form. To maintain confidentiality of the samples, whether a patient, staff member, or system function, codes known only to the data collector and the quality management council may be used. For many studies, however, in which confidentiality is not an issue, patients' identification numbers or staff members' employment numbers may be used. Note that for sample sizes greater than 20, an additional form or forms may be used.
12. Enter the indicator from the indicator development form. Since indicators take the form of a fraction or ratio, as a convenience to the data collector, the spaces in which to enter the numerator and denominator are clearly marked.

KEY
+ met
- did not meet
e exception

① Study Start Date: Jan 15, 1990
② Study End Date: Jan 25, 1990
③ Dept.: Oncology ④ Study Number: #157-A

⑤ Data Collectors:
1. Marilyn Dennison RN
2. Lois Wilkens RN
3. Cheryl Carbaugh RN

⑥ Important Aspect: Pain mgt. of Terminal Oncology Pt.

⑦ ☒ High Volume ☒ High Risk ☒ Problem Prone ☒ High Cost

⑧ Sample Size: 20 of 2.0*

⑨ Exceptions:
1. RN employed < 3 months
2. _____
3. _____

⑩ Remarks: Indicator B (Staff-process)
* Exceptions will be eliminated and sample size lowered.

⑪ Indicator

⑫ Number of oncology RNs ⑬
Numerator certified in pain control
Denominator total # of oncology RNs

	1-1	2-1	3-1	4-1	5-1	6-1	7-1	8-1	9-1	10-1	11-1	12-1	13-1	14-1	15-1	16-1	17-1	18-1	19-1	20-1	⑭ Totals +	-	e	⑮ Results %	⑯ Within Parameters Yes	No
	+	-	+	+	e	+	+	+	+	e	+	-	-	e	+	+	+	e	+		13	3	4	81%		✓

⑰ Demographic Data
RNs who have failed to achieve the 90% passing score on first try ✓

⑳ 19% failed to pass certification exam on first try

⑱ Demographic Data
RNs who took certification test twice ✓✓

㉑ 25% had to take the test twice to achieve the 90% passing score

⑲ Demographic Data
RNs who took certification test more than twice ✓

㉒ 12% had to repeat the test more than twice to achieve a passing score

■ FIGURE 9-1 Data collection form. (© 1991 Jackie Katz and Ellie Green. Reprinted with permission.)

13. Enter a + if the response is positive to the indicator, enter a − if the response is negative to the indicator, and enter an *e* for an exception. There is a space for each response per sample. The key is located in the upper right hand corner of the form.

14. These spaces are used to total the number of positive and negative responses to the indicator and the number of exceptions. Add and enter the number of positive responses. Add and enter the number of negative responses. Add and enter the number of exceptions. Subtract the number of exceptions from the total sample size. In the example shown there were four exceptions from a sample size of 20. Subtracting the four exceptions from the sample size of 20 leaves 16 in the sample.

15. This column is used to enter the percent of compliance. To calculate compliance divide the total number of positive responses by the adjusted (i.e., excluding exceptions) sample size of 16. In the example there were 13 positive responses; 13 divided by 16 equals 0.81 or 81%.

16. This column is used in conjunction with the threshold parameters determined on the indicator development form. If the data fall within the established threshold parameters, then the box marked "yes" is checked. If the data fall outside the established parameters, then the box marked "no" is checked.

17-19. Boxes 17 to 19 with their accompanying spaces permit data collectors to record relevant demographic data. Factors that may assist in the identification of patterns or trends when data analysis occurs are considered demographic data. In the example, data were collected about the number of oncology RNs certified in pain control management on the oncology unit. Demographic data include RNs who failed to achieve the 90% mandatory passing score on the first try.

20-22. These boxes are used for a brief analysis of the demographic data. In the example, 19% of the RNs failed to pass the certification exam on the first try. This additional information provides an extra dimension of thoroughness to the analysis. Demographic data may include the department, or the shift on which an incident occurred, or the nurse or physician involved. This portion may include information about the patient being studied, such as height, weight, sex, and room number. It may include any of the patient, staff, or system variables listed on the indicator development form.

QMC Tracking Form

In THE BLUEPRINT, a QMC tracking form is reproduced on the reverse side of the data collection form. Once the data collection has been completed by the department data collector, the data collection form is returned to the QMC, and their review and tracking are entered on the QMC tracking tool. This form is shown in Figure 9-2. Directions for use are as follows:

1. Copy the indicator from the data collection tool to avoid the necessity of flipping back and forth each time new information is entered.
2. Enter the date.
3. Enter the analysis of the initial monitoring in brief sentences.
4. If a justification of variance is required, check with the council which must make the justification and then route the form to it. Either the executive nurse council, clinical, professional, or administrative practice council will receive

① Indicator: ② Date:

③ I. Analysis of Initial Monitoring

④ *Recommendations:*

　　　　□ Justification of Variance required
　　　　　Route to:
　　　　　　□ Executive Nurse Council
　　　　　　□ Clinical Practice Council
　　　　　　□ Professional Practice Council
　　　　　　□ Administrative Practice Council

　　　　□ Continue Monitoring Plan

⑤ II. Justification

⑥ *Recommendations:*

　　　　□ No further action needed, continue monitoring plan
　　　　□ Additional review required
　　　　　　□ second reviewer
　　　　　　□ query review
　　　　　　□ intensive review

■ **FIGURE 9-2   QMC tracking form.**
(© 1991 Jackie Katz and Ellie Green. Reprinted with permission.)

the form and investigate the variance. If no justification is required check the box marked "continue monitoring plan."

5. This space is for the council, to whom the form was routed in step 4, to write a justification of the identified variance. This justification is returned to the QMC.

6. Recommendations are then made by the QMC based on its analysis of step 5. The QMC may decide that no further action is necessary, in which case monitoring will continue as planned. If the QMC decides that an additional review is necessary, it must check the type of review that is required—either a second reviewer opinion, a query review by a department or person, or an intensive review by an appropriate council.

Forms for Management Rounds

Figure 9-3 presents a simple form that may be used to collect data on administrative rounds. It consolidates information from a trifocus of patient, staff, and system. Once completed, it may be kept in a loose-leaf binder for easy reference. When an issue or concern repeatedly surfaces, this form helps to justify appropriate actions or expenditure of resources to solve the problem. No management round should exceed one half hour of the manager's time. For this reason the form is designed with space for interviewing a maximum of three staff members and three patients as well as space to make no more than three observations on any given round. The form is self-explanatory. It is especially useful for novice managers.

End-of-Shift Report

Figure 9-4 is an example of an end-of-shift report. This form is one of the most popular multidisciplinary data collection tools of THE BLUEPRINT. Used successfully by many hospitals, it provides concurrent, continuous, planned, organized data collection from all three sources—consumer, deliverer, and manager—in other words, the three domains. This end-of-shift report replaces the former "generic screen" monitors.

The end-of-shift report provides a method for continuous data collection about the happenings in each department within the division of nursing with relatively little effort. Blank copies (at least 21; one for each shift for 1 week) are hung on a clipboard in the nursing station in an area visible to all personnel. Nurses, physicians, supervisors, risk managers, infection control nurses, and others are not only encouraged to use the information on the report, but also are encouraged to add pertinent information.

It is the duty of the charge nurse to oversee the completion of the report at the end of his or her shift and replace it on the clipboard. The reports accumulate for the week. At the end of the week, the data are compiled by the department manager or the quality management coordinator. The information is tabulated and sent to QMC for divisional tracking.

One of the outstanding features of this end-of-shift report is the build-in tracking of "clinical outliers." "Clinical outlier" is a term coined by the authors to designate a patient care situation that extends beyond a time frame established by a multidisciplinary task force. Examples of clinical outliers include invasive devices such as IVs, arterial lines, Swan-Ganz catheters, staples, sutures, Foley catheters, endotracheal tubes, and so on which are not removed within the designated time frames. Once the

DATE _____ TIME _____ UNIT _____

STAFF MEMBERS INTERVIEWED	CONCERNS/ ACCOLADES	ACTIONS TO BE TAKEN	DATE OF ACTION
1. _____			
2. _____			
3. _____			

PATIENTS/SOs INTERVIEWED	CONCERNS/ ACCOLADES	ACTIONS TO BE TAKEN	DATE OF ACTION
1. _____			
2. _____			
3. _____			

MANAGER OBSERVATIONS	CONCERNS/ ACCOLADES	ACTIONS TO BE TAKEN	DATE OF ACTION
1. _____			
2. _____			
3. _____			

■ FIGURE 9-3   Management rounds quality assessment form.

1. Date: Shift: Department:

	Rm #/Classification	3. Admissions	4. Discharges	5. Problems related to:
2.	Surgeries (Reg):	Rm #/Class.	Rm #/Class.	1) Bed utilization:
				2) Physicians:
	Short Stays:			3) Equipment/Supplies:
				4) Assignments/Staff Members:
	Observations:			
				5) Patient/Family:

6.	Transferred to another facility:	
7.	Emergency Procedures/Codes/Deaths	8. Outstanding Employee:
		Why?
		9. Outstanding Physician:
		Why?

10. Pace/Workload: Quiet   Steady Busy   Very Busy   Short-staffed by acuity   Specify:

11. Report patients who: Name/Rm #

1. Develop a decubitus not present on admission
2. Have a decubitus present on admission
3. Develop Pulmonary Edema not present on admission
4. Develop CHF not present on admission
5. Aspirate within the hospital
6. Develop post-op respiratory problems
7. Develop IV complications
8. Fall/Injuries
9. Temps > 100° F
10. Develop post-op wound infection
11. Hemorrhage

12. Also report department clinical outliers

1.
2.
3.
4.

13. Comments:

14. Signature(s):

■ **FIGURE 9-4   The end-of-shift report.**
(© 1991 Roane General Hospital. Reprinted with permission.)

multidisciplinary task force completes its list of clinical outlier time frames, the list is posted in every nurses' station beside the end-of-shift report. When an invasive device remains in a patient beyond the time frame established by the task force, the patient is listed on the end-of-shift report as a clinical outlier. It is the duty of the charge nurse to list each outlier and the duty of the attending physician or RN to justify or explain the reason for the extended use of the device on the clinical outlier justification tool on the reverse side of the end-of-shift report. Figure 9-5 shows the justification tool that is printed on the reverse side of the end-of-shift report. Since there are no national guidelines to direct the multidisciplinary task force in creating clinical outliers, each organization's task force must establish guidelines for its own use. Some specialty organizations and some manufacturers may have suggested guidelines that might prove helpful to the task force.

The end-of-shift report obviates the need for occurrence or generic screening because nothing "slips through the cracks" when this method is used. In fact, it not only becomes one of the organization's most valuable data collection tools, but also can save the organization hundreds of dollars each year in setting up and carrying out monitoring and evaluation studies. Numerous small studies are unnecessary when the data are being collected already on every shift in every department in the organization.

The QMC may use the data from each department's end-of-shift report to create a division-wide picture of the quality of care. Using this ongoing data collection method assures that the QMC will have concurrent information that will alert it to any adverse trends and allow it to take immediate remedial action.

Here are the directions for using the end-of-shift report. The numbers on the form correspond to the following numbered explanations.

1. Enter the date, shift, and department.
2. In the spaces in this column, list the room number and acuity classification for the surgeries that occur during the shift, the patients who are admitted during the shift for a short stay, and those admitted for observation.
3. Enter the routine admissions to the department by room number and acuity classification.
4. Enter the room number and acuity classification of the patients discharged from the department during this shift.
5. Enter a brief description of each problem related to:
   a. Bed utilization—problems such as boarding patients in the emergency department because beds are filled to capacity, and difficulty transferring patients to another area, are examples of bed utilization problems that should be noted.
   b. Physicians—when physicians have problems locating supplies, or make requests for special instruments or equipment, or have a dissatisfaction with anyone or anything within the department, it should be noted in this space.
   c. Equipment and supplies—all broken equipment or missing supplies from the department should be noted.
   d. Assignments and staff members—reasons for refusing an assignment should be noted. Any staff member problem such as an injury, or leaving the department owing to sudden illness, or emergency should be recorded in this space.
   e. Patient or family—any problems relating directly to the patient or the family should be noted in this space. Examples include a family that is abusive to patient or staff, and a patient who habitually screams, attempts to get out of bed, or is combative.

JUSTIFICATION
OF CLINICAL OUTLIERS

DEPT ______________________

SHIFT ______________________

DATE ______________________

Key

1 - acceptable noncompliance no recommendations
2 - acceptable noncompliance with recommendations
3 - unacceptable noncompliance

			RATING		
PATIENT	CLINICAL OUTLIERS	JUSTIFICATION BY MD/RN	1	2	3

■ **FIGURE 9-5 Justification tool.**
(© 1991 Jackie Katz and Ellie Green. Reprinted with permission.)

6. Enter the name of any patient who is transferred to another facility during this shift.

7. List any emergency procedures, codes, or deaths that occur on this shift. Also, enter the patient's name and room number.

8. Enter the name of any staff member who exhibited outstanding behavior during this shift. Explain why this behavior was so appreciated by the other staff members.

9. Enter the name of any physician who extended himself or herself on behalf of the nursing staff during this shift. Explain why the physician's behavior was appreciated.

10. This space is used to track the pace of the department. Any shift that is not staffed correctly by acuity should be noted on the end-of-shift report. This information can be used to justify the need for increased staffing.

11. Enter the names and room numbers of all patients who exhibit any of the indicators listed. This section of the end-of-shift report is used to track division-wide indicators. Each individual department submits the information to the division of nursing QMC for comparison and evaluation. QMC uses such continuously collected data to create an overall analysis of the care and service within the organization.

12. List in this section department clinical outliers as they occur on each shift. Use the list created by the multidisciplinary task force that is posted in the department.

13. Add comments that help explain any of the collected data in this space. Important comments from families or patients may also be noted in this space.

14. The charge nurse who is responsible for this shift for the report should sign his or her name in this space.

This end-of-shift report has proven valuable to many organizations in collecting concurrent data. It may, of course, be adapted to suit any department or situation. It provides a tool for ongoing, continuous, organized, planned, systematic data collection in health care organizations.

Suggestion Boxes

Every health care organization should establish some means of open communication with visitors, staff members, physicians, vendors; in short, anyone from within or outside the organization who has a problem, suggestion, or desire to communicate information with the organization's administration. To foster communication, suggestion boxes can be prominently displayed in highly visible areas and suggestions can be solicited from all three sources of data: the consumer, the deliverer, and management.

Shady Grove Adventist Hospital in Rockville, Maryland established a very successful suggestion system called "The Sounding Board." The "Sounding Board" form shown in Figure 9-6 is visible in a plastic container near every elevator in the building. A sign encourages all who pass by to share constructive suggestions and comments with the administration of the hospital. Commitments are made to maintain confidentiality and to channel the question to the person in the organization who can best answer it. A personal interview may also be scheduled upon request. The organization reports that many, both staff and visitors, take advantage of this forum for communicating with the administration.

SOUNDING BOARD

Sounding Board provides opportunity for you, as an employee of Shady Grove Adventist Hospital, to have a voice—to "sound-off" about any subject related to your work specifically, or the hospital program in general.

We encourage constructive suggestions and comments, and will attempt to answer in complete confidence *bonafide* complaints or criticism regarding policies or problems. No one knows your name except the Sounding Board manager, who will channel your question to the one who can best answer it. All replies will be returned directly to you.

If you request a personal interview, Sounding Board will arrange the appointment in strict confidence.

Please use a separate
form for each subject.   Date _____

Comments: _____

_____

_____

_____

_____

☐ Check here if you want to discuss your comments or questions
   with a qualified person.

Name _____

Home address _____

Job title _____

Department _____

Sounding Board needs this information only to forward your reply. If you do not include your name and address, we will not know where to send the answer to your question.

COMPLETED FORM MAY BE SENT BY HOSPITAL INTERMAIL OR POSTAL SERVICE.

■ **FIGURE 9-6** **"Sounding board"** form.
(Used with permission of Shady Grove Adventist Hospital, Rockville, MD.)

Dear Former Patient

Recently, we were privileged to serve you as a patient at Ballard Community Hospital. We would appreciate your assistance in evaluating our services by taking a few minutes to express your thoughts regarding your stay in the hospital on this short questionnaire.

Thank you for helping us to continue to improve and thereby serve you and others more effectively.

Sincerely,

Administrator

(Please circle ONE number for each item)

ADMITTING/REGISTRATION	Needs Improvement			Excellent		Does Not Apply
1. Waiting time before admission processing	1	2	3	4	5	____
2. Thoroughness in answering questions, explaining forms and procedures	1	2	3	4	5	____
3. Courtesy and efficiency of admitting process	1	2	3	4	5	____

Comments _____

ROOM ACCOMMODATIONS	Needs Improvement			Excellent		Does Not Apply
4. Decor of your room	1	2	3	4	5	____
5. Cleanliness of your room	1	2	3	4	5	____
6. Temperature of your room	1	2	3	4	5	____
7. Quietness of your room	1	2	3	4	5	____
8. Telephone service	1	2	3	4	5	____

Comments _____

NURSING SERVICE	Needs Improvement			Excellent		Does Not Apply
9. Was your admission to your room handled in a courteous, efficient manner?	1	2	3	4	5	____
10. Were you made comfortable within your first few hours here?	1	2	3	4	5	____
11. Did the nursing staff give prompt attention to your needs and requests?	1	2	3	4	5	____
12. Did the nursing staff explain your hospital routine adequately?	1	2	3	4	5	____
13. Were you taught how to care for yourself after leaving the hospital?	1	2	3	4	5	____

Comments _____

SPECIAL TESTS AND PROCEDURES	Needs Improvement			Excellent		Does Not Apply
14. Were tests explained to you so that you were prepared for what was going to happen?	1	2	3	4	5	____
15. Was enough time allowed for you to ask questions?	1	2	3	4	5	____

Comments _____

NUTRITION/FOOD SERVICE	Needs Improvement			Excellent		Does Not Apply
16. Were you put on a special diet? If so, what type?	1 - Yes			2 - No		
17. Attractiveness and taste of food	1	2	3	4	5	____
Hot food served hot	1	2	3	4	5	____
Cold food served cold	1	2	3	4	5	____
18. Variety and selection of food items	1	2	3	4	5	____
19. Receiving the food items ordered	1	2	3	4	5	____
20. If you received nutritional information from a dietitian, was it useful and meaningful?	1	2	3	4	5	____

Comments _____

VISITORS	Needs Improvement			Excellent		Does Not Apply
21. Helpfulness of the hospital staff and volunteers to your visitors	1	2	3	4	5	____
22. Convenience of the visiting hours for family and friends	1	2	3	4	5	____

Comments _____

SIGNS AND DIRECTIONS	Needs Improvement			Excellent		Does Not Apply
23. Signs and directions outside the hospital	1	2	3	4	5	____
24. Signs and directions inside the hospital	1	2	3	4	5	____

Comments _____

■ **FIGURE 9-7** Patient satisfaction survey example.
(© 1991 Ballard Community Hospital, Seattle, WA. Reprinted with permission.)

PARKING

	Needs Improvement			Excellent		Does Not Apply
25. Convenience of parking	1	2	3	4	5	_____
26. Directions to parking	1	2	3	4	5	_____

Comments _____
_____
_____

PATIENT BILLING/CREDIT DEPARTMENT

	Needs Improvement			Excellent		Does Not Apply
27. If you talked with the billing/credit dept., were you given a satisfactory explanation of charges and insurance coverage?....................................	1	2	3	4	5	_____
28. Cooperation of the hospital in arranging your payment	1	2	3	4	5	_____

Comments _____
_____
_____

STAFF

		Needs Improvement			Excellent		Does Not Apply
29. How were you treated by the other staff members you came in contact with?							
	A. Physicians	1	2	3	4	5	_____
	B. Admissions	1	2	3	4	5	_____
	C. Emergency Department	1	2	3	4	5	_____
	D. Physical Therapy....................................	1	2	3	4	5	_____
	E. Laboratory	1	2	3	4	5	_____
	F. Respiratory Care Dept.	1	2	3	4	5	_____
	G. Housekeeping......................................	1	2	3	4	5	_____
	H. X-Ray	1	2	3	4	5	_____
	I. Transportation.....................................	1	2	3	4	5	_____
	J. Volunteers	1	2	3	4	5	_____
	K. Business Office	1	2	3	4	5	_____
	L. EKG/EEG	1	2	3	4	5	_____
	M. Hospital Telephone Operator...........................	1	2	3	4	5	_____
	N. Others _____	1	2	3	4	5	_____
	Specify						

GOING HOME

	Needs Improvement			Excellent		Does Not Apply
30. Please rate Ballard Community Hospital on an OVERALL basis for the service and care we gave. Please circle only one number...................................	1	2	3	4	5	_____
31. Would you choose Ballard Community Hospital again?	1 - Yes			2 - No		_____

32. Please list the things you liked during your stay at Ballard Community Hospital.
_____
_____
_____

33. Please list the things you liked least during your stay at Ballard Community Hospital.
_____
_____
_____

34. Who completed the questionnaire:
    1 - Patient   2 - Family Member   3 - Friend

35. Additional comments or suggestions:
_____
_____
_____

PATIENT PROFILE

36. Please complete the general information below:

Date of Discharge _____
        Month   Day   Year

Room # _____

Length of Stay: _____   A. 1 day
                             B. 2 - 3 days
                             C. 4 - 6 days
                             D. 1 - 2 weeks
                             E. Over 2 weeks (14 days or more)

Your age category: _____   A. 18 - 24
                                 B. 25 - 34
                                 C. 35 - 44
                                 D. 45 - 54
                                 E. 55 - 64
                                 F. 65 - 74
                                 G. 75 and over

37. Do you want to be contacted by a hospital representative to further discuss your hospitalization ....   1 - Yes   2 - No

If yes, please note telephone number and best time(s) to call:

(   )
Area Code   Telephone Number   Time(s) to call

_____
                            Name

Your sex is _____   A. Female   B. Male

Thank you for your cooperation in completing this questionnaire. Should you desire to remain anonymous, please remove address label and do not sign your name.

No postage required.

THANK YOU.

■ **FIGURE 9-7, cont'd.**

Satisfaction Surveys

It is critical that health care organizations establish adequate measures of patient satisfaction with their care and services. There must be an effective means for quickly identifying complaints and problems. The satisfaction of all three of the domains is vital to a well-rounded quality management program.

An example of a patient satisfaction survey from Ballard Community Hospital in Seattle, Washington, appears in Figure 9-7. Once the questionnaire is developed and distributed to patients, it must be treated as a serious method of data collection. The data must be compiled and used to create change and improvement within the organization.

Staff and administrative satisfaction surveys are useful mechanisms for evaluating the professional and management morale, a major factor in retention. These surveys may be formal or informal. They can be conducted by outside consultants or developed internally. Information can be gathered from questionnaires, in individual counseling sessions, or in group discussions.

Hot Lines

Many health care organizations have found that establishing a "hot line" works well to keep them informed of problems or complaints. Some organizations offer inpatients a phone number to call to discuss any problem, question, or gripe. Such hot lines are usually staffed by patient representatives. They serve the important function of defusing acute dissatisfaction while the patient is still in the hospital and experiencing it.

Administration, from the first line manager to the chief executive officer, may also have a hot line or open phone policy whereby any staff member may call to discuss a problem or issue. These hot lines can eliminate paperwork and save the time and frustration involved in reaching the right person fast.

Focus Groups

Focus groups can also serve as an excellent mechanism for collecting information. Focus groups are an assembly of a representative sample of patient, staff, or administrators brought together to discuss a particular quality problem or opportunity.

Patient focus groups, in particular, are an essential data gathering device.[2] In these groups, recent former patients exchange opinions and comments on their hospital experience. Such focus groups provide narrative compliments and complaints to expand upon information gathered through questionnaires. This feedback helps staff members identify and solve specific problems. Former patients are usually delighted and flattered when asked to participate in such sessions.[2]

Staff and management groups may also be assembled for fact finding. In addition, a portion of staff and management meetings may be used for the purpose of collecting data regarding specific, important aspects of professional or administrative service.

The importance of accurate, meaningful data collection cannot be overstated. It is only through gathering and analyzing facts that meaningful change and improvement can occur in health care organizations. Errors and incidents will always occur. While important, they can be, nevertheless, the cause of "knee jerk" reactions that waste resources and solve few problems. Health care organizations can avoid knee jerk reactions to problems and subsequent wasted resources through the creation and management of sound systems that collect, organize, and react to data in a planned, organized, systematic way.

REFERENCES

1. Juran JM: Juran's quality control handbook, ed 4, New York, 1988, McGraw Hill Book Co.
2. The Law, Medicine, and Health Care 12(2): 53-62, 1984.
3. Walton M: The Deming management method, New York, 1986, Putnam Publishing Co.
4. Walton M: Deming management at work, New York, 1990, Putnam Publishing Co.

10

STEP 7:
EVALUATING VARIATION

*Ignorance of variation lies at the root
of many problems in health care.*

RAFAEL AGUAYO

Kay Waldo, nurse manager of a 45-bed medical unit, was puzzled. Another patient had developed a pressure ulcer. What was the cause of the increasing occurrence of pressure ulcers in her unit? Silently she stood looking at the sleeping 84-year-old patient who was her department's latest victim of "alterations in skin integrity" and wondered how he had developed the ulceration on his buttocks so quickly.

"This is the ninth case this month," she mused. "That will blow our department's statistical control this quarter for skin integrity and I'll be outside of my threshold parameters." She walked slowly back to her office thinking, "This is certainly a special cause variation and it will have to be justified. If I try to fix it, will I be tampering? I want to make sure that the incidence of hospital-acquired pressure ulcers in this department is rare, even if it is a rate-based indicator! I will have to decide on one of the scientific tools, gather my staff, and get busy. I can't tolerate a variance like this."

Nurse Waldo was using a thought process and language that is increasingly common among health care professionals. Words like statistical control, variance, special cause variation, threshold parameters, and tampering describe a scientific approach to quality management that is revolutionizing quality concepts. Although these words may be new to many health care quality professionals, they are not difficult to understand. While many statistical concepts are quite sophisticated, the implications of the few covered in this chapter are simple. Before we explore these concepts, we'll consider the forces that are creating the shift to statistically based approaches to quality management.

Driving the revolutionary change are two forces: the Joint Commission and the increasing cost of health care. When the Joint Commission listed "evaluate the variation" as step 7 of the ten-step process, an interest was kindled among quality professionals in the subject of "variance." They began to ask, "What is variance and how does it apply to our role in quality management?" Variation was also seen as the "cause" and "cure" of increased health care costs.

No longer are quality management professionals praised for writing lengthy, narrative quarterly reports of happenings in their departments with suggested corrective actions based on their own hunches, experience, or opinions. Rather, they are expected to use a scientific approach to problem solving and thus generate true improvement. Why the necessity for a scientific approach?

"It's simple," says Barbara Sines, RN, MSN, acting manager of surgical services at Washington Adventist Hospital in Takoma Park, Maryland. "We can no longer afford 'experimental' health care. We must place our management, care delivery and appraisal practices on a scientific basis to prevent wasted resources. Furthermore, we need to educate our staff so that they can develop problem solving strategies that are rooted in the scientific process. When we do, staff members will find solutions that work the first time. Costs will drop and the quality of care will improve."[8] In other words, Ms. Sines is opposed to a trial and error management style that wastes resources. She recognizes that problem-solving mechanisms that "work the first time" reduce costs by conserving resources and effectively managing staff, equipment, and supplies.

■ THE SCIENTIFIC APPROACH

"The core of quality improvement methods is summed up in two words: scientific approach."[7] A scientific approach is simply a systematic, planned, organized method for problem solving that is understood and followed by all employees. Decisions to act are based on data rather than experience, hunches, or "gut" feelings. The scientific approach ensures that an organization will search for the root cause of a problem, "smoke it out" and fix it, rather than implement a quick, short-term, "knee-jerk" fix. Just as a band-aid may temporarily hide a malignant mole, so a "band-aid fix" may hide a problem within a health care organization—for a time. Sooner or later, however, the "band-aid" will be insufficient to hide the greater problem. It is more cost effective and better for the health of the individual and institution to address the real cause of the problem. Fixing the cause may sometimes be difficult. It may require rethinking your health care organization's current approach to quality. It may also necessitate committing sufficient resources to quality improvement (QI).

However, a willingness to alter the present position and commit resources does not by itself ensure QI. In addition, a scientific approach must be instituted if QI is to become a reality.

Implementing this approach may require changing some of our long-held QA concepts because QI cannot occur in the traditional environment. QI involves adopting a trifocus approach to monitoring and evaluation. In other words, when a problem or quality opportunity occurs, the organization will look at every aspect of that problem or opportunity—not just at nursing care—to identify ways to achieve QI.

"What goes on in nursing care—even the outcomes of nursing care—are not the result of just what nurses do," says Paul M. Schyve, MD, the Joint Commission's vice president for research and standards. "All of the processes [within a health care organization] affect outcomes." To affect the probability of good outcomes, he added, hospitals must "study those processes intensely, then improve the processes."[5]

■ WHAT ARE THE PROCESSES IN A HEALTH CARE ORGANIZATION?

Processes in a health care organization refer to all of the patient, staff, and system activities that occur. Examples of processes include admitting and discharging a patient; delivering medication to a patient; transferring a patient to another area; carrying out a surgical procedure; performing tests on a patient; managing pain, infection control, patient safety; and the like. All of these processes involve multiple care givers within the organization. If this were a perfect world, all processes would be error-free and all providers would be perfect. Unfortunately, health care organizations operate in an imperfect world with imperfect human providers. For that reason, variations in processes occur. "One may seek to minimize variation by eliminating sources of variation, but variations will never be eliminated entirely."[9] The effort to do so results in continuous improvement.

■ VARIATIONS

There are two kinds of variations. The first is called common cause variance.[2] This involves the minor variations that occur within a health care organization regardless of how excellent the program is. Often, they can be changed only by management. Common cause variations may include minor variations in a staff member's abilities, an unclear procedure, limitations of equipment, and the like. Because resources are unavailable to detect the cause of every minor variation, they are tolerated. In addition, many variations are caused by chance. When chance is the cause of a variation it would be futile to investigate the cause and try to fix it. Variations caused by chance are tolerated.

Organizations that do not recognize the chance phenomenon spend much time, effort, and money investigating variations in their system that could not be altered even if the reasons for them were found. Unfortunately, often employees are blamed. It is thought that if employees would only try harder, be more efficient, work together, and be more loyal, every variance would vanish. Organizations implement elaborate mechanisms designed to educate, test, and exhort employees only to find that no improvement occurs. Employees may already be working as hard as they can and minor variations caused by chance cannot be "fixed."

The phenomenon of chance within an organization and the futility of blaming employees for variations in process has been demonstrated by Dr. Deming in his famous red bead experiment.[9] In this exercise, Dr. Deming demonstrates the need to use acceptable parameters instead of absolute thresholds as a benchmark for the evaluation of processes.

Here is the exercise: Dr. Deming chooses six members of the audience. He tells them he is recruiting them to be trained to work in his factory. He appoints two of them inspectors and one chief inspector. Deming serves as the foreman. The remaining three serve as the "workers."

This factory, Dr. Deming explains, makes white beads. Occasionally, however, it turns out red beads. The red beads are defective. The company only gets paid for white beads.

Dr. Deming instructs the workers to scoop up the white beads from one of two pans containing a mixture of white and red beads in a ratio of 4 white to 1 red. A rectangular paddle with 50 holes is used to scoop the beads and workers are expected to achieve no more than 2 red beads per scoop. The threshold for noncompliance is 4%.

Each paddleful must be reviewed by an inspector who counts the number of red beads. This is verified by the chief inspector who announces the count and dismisses the worker.

After the first try, a performance review is conducted. Each worker then makes three more scooping attempts. Again, after each scoop, a performance review is conducted. The results vary; a different worker achieves the best and worst results with each try. The performance of each worker varies from scoop to scoop purely by chance! There is a variation among the workers ranging from a low of 4 red beads to a high of 18—all by chance.

Most of us assume chance plays a minor role in variations in the performance of individual workers. However, here is a case where chance is responsible for 100% of it. Suppose that management eliminates the workers with the poorest performance and keeps the top three workers. The workers with low error rates must complete two more attempts each. Once again chance comes into play and the results reflect it. In this case, the three best workers produce the worst overall performance in the company's history! "When all the variation in performance is due to chance, past performance is neither a guarantee nor an indication of future performance."[1]

In the bead factory example, individuals were held accountable for variations in their performance that were, in fact, caused by the system. They had no control over their level of performance.

The second kind of variation is called special cause variance.[2] Special cause variations occur when systems and processes break down. There are several possible reasons for process breakdowns, such as employee error, lack of knowledge of the process, and breakdown of equipment. Special causes are usually easier to correct than common causes. Setting threshold parameters makes it possible to identify special cause variations while tolerating common cause fluctuations.

An organization must have a scientific method for distinguishing between common cause and special cause variation. That scientific method is statistical control.

■ STATISTICAL CONTROL OF PROCESSES

In order to function effectively and efficiently, health care organizations must maintain statistical control of their processes. When an organization knows that it is in statistical control, it can be confident of its outcomes and begin to work toward quality improvement.

The term statistical control may be new to many health care quality professionals but it describes a simple concept. Statistical control means that things are happening the way they were planned to happen—that is, the results fall within the threshold parameters, predetermined by the organization. When a process within the organization is in statistical control it is referred to as a stable system.[2]

In his research, Dr. Deming has demonstrated that when a variation is caused by chance, almost all of the data will fall within three standard deviations from the average.[10] Within a stable system, variations occur within predetermined parameters. The parameters, or upper and lower limits of the range, are the control limits (threshold parameters). These control limits are set by the quality professional. When all the collected data fall within the control limits, the system is considered stable, i.e., in statistical control. Variations that fall within the control limits are assumed to be caused by chance.

Figure 10-1 is an example of a control chart that tracks the incidence of urinary tract infections within 72 hours following insertion of a Foley catheter in a 640-bed medical center. Based on historical data, parameters have been set with the lower control limit at 30 and the upper control limit at 50.

When a result falls above or below the control limits, it is out of control. Figure 10-2 shows a control chart that demonstrates a variation out of control. When this happens, an immediate analysis of the variation is warranted. Variations outside of the control limits are called special cause variations and should be investigated.

Chance cannot be eliminated from the system. Special circumstances, however, can be corrected. For example, some patients enter hospitals with urinary tract infec-

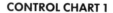

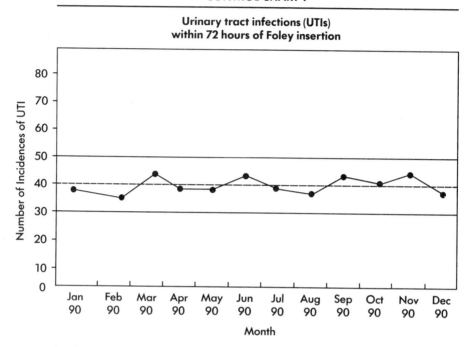

INFORMATION FOR 1990
COMPILATION OF DATA FROM ALL DEPARTMENTS

■ FIGURE 10-1   Control Chart 1—urinary tract infections.

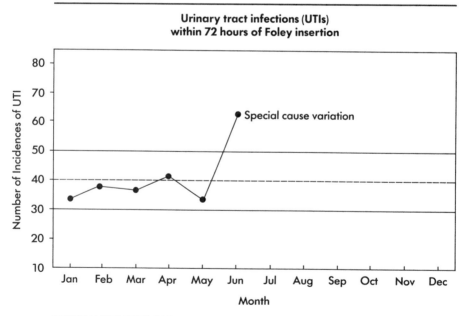

INFORMATION FOR 1991

■ FIGURE 10-2   Control Chart 2—urinary tract infections.

tions (UTIs), unbeknownst to the patient, the physician, or nurse. Therefore, it is unrealistic to blame staff members for all urinary tract infections occurring in catheterized patients. However, a sudden rise in the incidence of UTIs is a special cause variance, and it must be investigated. Likewise, results that are better than expected should also be investigated to confirm reliability in the data collection process.

A system that is in statistical control is not necessarily ideal or defect-free. Rather, the system is stable and any problem may be attacked at its "root." Until statistical control is achieved, no real work can begin to find solutions to special cause variations in processes.

Furthermore, once statistical control is achieved for a process, improvement in that process can only be achieved through a change in the system—not a change in individual workers. Statistical control helps people stop needless searching for special causes when there is only a minor variation in results. It also eliminates unnecessary action to attempt to improve minor variations. Thus it controls the costs associated with improvement efforts by eliminating the possibility of tampering. Initiating corrective action aimed at improving staff performance will not result in any appreciable change in the variance and may distort the results of the next study. Also, these attempts to improve staff performance may waste scarce resources that are needed to improve the true cause of the variation.

■ TAMPERING WITH STABLE PROCESSES

Typically, when variations arise in the results of a monitoring study, there is an attempt to resolve the cause of the variation by changing/correcting the process. However, attempts to correct minor shifts within the threshold parameters may, in fact, produce worse results. Attempting to fix one part of a process distorts the other parts. As the problems resulting from the distortion start to surface, more and more steps are added to compensate.[7] This is called tampering. Tampering is a "knee jerk" correction in response to a variation in study results, whether the results are due to common or special causes. Tampering creates wildly fluctuating variations in processes that, in turn, yield meaningless data as a benchmark against which to measure progress.

Often when a process varies, health care professionals' trying to fix it causes another fluctuation in data. More tampering is then necessary to correct what appears to be a greater problem. Tampering with a stable system is not productive, because it typically results in overcorrecting or undercorrecting the problem. Each correction may cost the organization thousands of dollars with no improvement noted in the processes, creating a lot of frustration in employees. The constant upheaval within the organization results in a great deal of motion but little direction. No sound improvements can occur from unstable, unexplainable, fluctuating data. Sound improvements can only occur in a stable system. As quality expert Rafael Aguayo says, "Ignorance of variation lies at the root of many problems in health care."[1]

One way for an organization to determine if tampering exists within their system is to look at the data being gathered. If it presents a roller coaster pattern, tampering is probably occurring.

When faced with negative data about outcomes of care, practice, or governance within an organization, it is easy to assume that each negative bit of information is due to one specific cause, such as the lack of effort of the staff member or poor clinical skills of the practitioner. The way to correct the situation, many reason, is to initiate new competency checks; test staff members; implement new programs; and exhort, bribe, or, perhaps, threaten staff members with the possibility of disciplinary action.

Having chosen one or more of these methods to enforce compliance, the monitoring of staff members becomes intense. It is reasoned that the data will show that improvements have resulted from these efforts.

Even some of our nation's most prestigious regulatory organizations mandate efforts to "tighten up the ship." For example, the Health Care Financing Administration (HCFA) has proposed a regulation requiring organizations to certify that their professional staff is competent to perform a guaiac test on patient's stool and to perform a finger stick for machine analysis of blood glucose levels. Yet, these tests may be purchased over the counter in any drug store and performed at home. Dennis O'Leary, MD, President of the Joint Commission, comments on HCFA's proposal this way, "To characterize HCFA's proposed regulations as onerous is an understatement. HCFA had an opportunity to introduce a modicum of sanity into the statutory requirements, but such rationality was apparently not within the agency's bag of surprises this time."[6]

Inherent in HCFA's proposal is the assumption that "correcting" the employee will correct the problem. Correcting only the employee, however, instead of the system may lead to tampering and unbalance a system that is already in statistical control.

Quality professionals must be alert to and avoid possible tampering. It can destabilize the system and create new problems that absorb the organization's resources. It accomplishes little and is difficult to stop.

An organization can improve and avoid tampering by first creating a stable system and then by eliminating special cause variations.

■ CREATING A STABLE SYSTEM

Creating a stable system requires tracking monitoring results of each aspect of care/service over time. The threshold parameter form shown in Figure 10-3 may be used to provide a visual display tracking of processes. Kay Waldo used the form to track the incidence of pressure ulcers in her department. Her threshold parameters were 0 to 4%. Upper and lower limits were marked on the graph. At the completion of each monthly study, data were entered on the graph to see if it fell within the threshold parameters. As long as the data fell within the threshold parameters of 0 to 4%, statistical control was maintained. When the data fell outside of the parameters, as it did in May, this was a signal for an immediate review.

When tracking data, the quality professional should realize that just being within the established parameters is not always sufficient to maintain quality. If data abruptly alter or show a marked trend, the system is also considered out of control—even when the data fall within established limits. Whenever the system is out of control, there is cause for immediate investigation. Ishikawa's *Guide to Quality Control* specifically states that a run chart is in statistical control when "1) All the points are within the control limits, and 2) The point grouping does not assume a particular form."[4] In other words, statistical control is achieved when the data fall within the preestablished parameters in a random pattern around the mean.

Figure 10-4 shows a threshold parameter form for a system that may be out of control even though the data remain within the established parameters. This study concerns the number of physicians' orders transcribed incorrectly. A 10% to 30% threshold, with a mean of 20%, has been established. (Note that in this case the mean *compliance* is 80%.) One glance at the graph shows that the system may be out of control even though the data fall within the control limits. It is also possible that the data will form an oscillating pattern and will come back down or it may indicate the

STUDY NUMBER _79-4007_ INDICATOR NUMBER _#3_
PRIMARY DATA COLLECTOR _Kay Waldo_
THRESHOLD PARAMETERS _0 - 4 %_

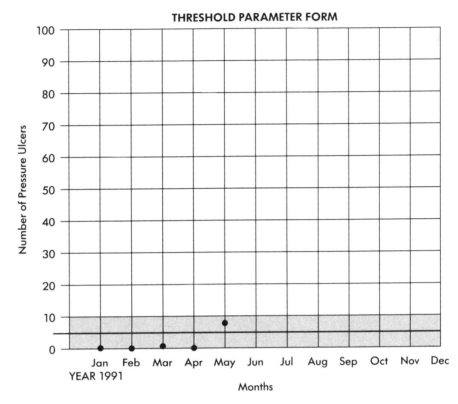

THRESHOLD PARAMETER FORM

Number of Pressure Ulcers (y-axis: 0, 10, 20, 30, 40, 50, 60, 70, 80, 90, 100)

Jan Feb Mar Apr May Jun Jul Aug Sep Oct Nov Dec
YEAR 1991

Months

REMARKS:

1. _No ulcers in this department this month (Jan.)_

2. _No ulcers in this department This month (Feb.)_

3. _One ulcer in This department which is on buttocks of 93-year-old incontinent pt. from extended care facility_

4. _No ulcers in this department this month_

5. _There are 9 pressure ulcers in This department This month. Investigation is underway._

6.

7.

8.

9.

10.

11.

12.

■ **FIGURE 10-3** Threshold parameter form for pressure ulcers.
(© 1991 Jackie Katz and Ellie Green. Reprinted with permission.)

STUDY NUMBER _87-999_ _____ INDICATOR NUMBER _#1_ _____
PRIMARY DATA COLLECTOR _Kim Young_ _____
THRESHOLD PARAMETERS _10-30 % (mean 20%)_ _____

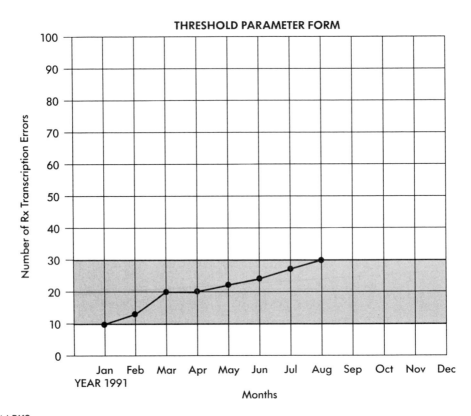

THRESHOLD PARAMETER FORM

REMARKS:

1. _Ten charts had Rx errors in transcription (see "folder" for breakdown)_
2. _Problem continues - discussed with charge nurses._
3. _Problem unabated. Spoke with Nurse Manager_
4. _Problem stabilized_
5. _Problem worsened. Called meeting with charge nurses and nurse managers_
6. _Problem worsened. Discussed at QMC._
7. _Discussed problem with Director of Nurses and Nurse Manager._
8. _Problem cannot be tolerated. Will call general meeting and discuss system of noting orders._
9.
10.
11.
12.

■ **FIGURE 10-4** Threshold parameter form for Rx transcription errors.
(© 1991 Jackie Katz and Ellie Green. Reprinted with permission.)

beginning of a long trend which may continue in an "out of control" pattern. In either event, an analysis must be done to determine the cause.

The upper and lower control limits are determined by allowing a process to run untampered and then analyzing the results. Refer to the process for setting thresholds described in Chapter 8. Every process has variations, but the more finely tuned the process, the less deviation there is from the average.

This is the reason for standardization of structure, outcome, process, and evaluation standards within THE BLUEPRINT. Good standards eliminate much of the variance inherent in any division of nursing. Once "roller coaster" variations are eliminated and a stable system is achieved, the organization can direct its resources toward improving the system.

■ ELIMINATING SPECIAL CAUSE VARIATIONS

A system can only be improved when special causes have been eliminated and the system has been brought into statistical control. Special cause variations can often be eliminated by workers just by virtue of creating awareness of the problem. For example, compliance to handwashing routine may improve dramatically when staff are aware that handwashing is being monitored. Action planning is the key to eliminating special cause variations and is described in Chapter 11.

■ STATISTICAL PROCESS CONTROL

Analysis of variations is accomplished through the use of specific tools designed to identify variation and to pinpoint causative factors. These tools are called statistical process control (SPC) tools. These tools are merely organized methods for describing problems and planning solutions. They help an individual or group to focus attention on a critical process of the organization that is causing difficulty, mentally "take it apart," look at it from every aspect, suggest methods to eliminate the difficulty, test the suggested methods, and then implement a permanent solution.

"Understanding quality leadership is not just rethinking where you are going," suggests Peter R. Scholtes, "it's looking at how you will get there. Paying attention to method as well as results is one of the distinguishing features of this new way [scientific approach] of doing business."[7] In other words, a scientific approach is necessary to move from the traditional methods of QA to the new approaches of QI.

In fact, Carole H. Patterson, MN, associate director of interpretation in the Joint Commission's department of standards recently pointed out, "The new nursing standards were revised to focus on a hospitalwide commitment to quality improvement."[5] If there is to be a hospital-wide commitment to quality, then QI must have a global focus within the organization with every aspect of care, practice, and governance coming under scrutiny.

Rewriting the standards, says Paul M. Schyve, MD, the Joint Commission's vice president for research and standards, is just the beginning of "the Joint Commission's attempt to move hospitals away from traditional quality assurance into QI."[5] Moving *from* QA *into* QI cannot be accomplished without a knowledge of scientific tools for decision making. A movement to the use of SPC tools in a health care organization entails a new way of looking at old situations. It requires an organization to look at every process affecting care, practice, and governance to see how those processes are carried out and how they can be improved. Schyve further states that finding oppor-

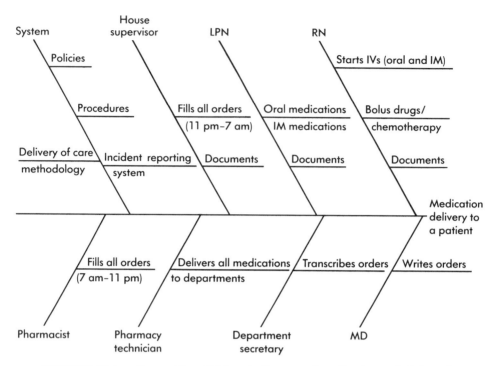

■ FIGURE 10-5   Cause-effect (fishbone) diagram of medications administration
to a patient.

tunities to improve nursing care does not mean simply focusing on nurses. In the past, Schyve notes, "QA activities often have attempted to determine: Did nurse A do the right thing? Did nurse B do the right thing?"[5] There was little need for a scientific approach when the focus of traditional QA activities was so narrow.

While there are many SPC tools that have been developed, some simple tools that may be used by quality professionals in the decision-making process are the fishbone diagram, flow chart, histogram, pareto chart, run chart, and control chart.

The cause and effect diagram—also known as the "fishbone" diagram because of its shape or the Ishikawa diagram after its originator, Kaoru Ishikawa—is used in brainstorming sessions to examine every factor that may influence a given situation. For example, the process of administration of medication from physician's order to delivery to a patient involves many people and departments. Figure 10-5 is an example of a cause and effect (fishbone) diagram that might be used in a problem-solving discussion focused on medication delivery.

The flow chart is an extremely useful way of analyzing what is happening. One way to begin is to determine the way a process actually works. Diagramming the process can immediately turn up redundancy, inefficiency, and misunderstanding.

For example, a flow chart of the process of same day surgery is shown in Figure 10-6. Is the patient flow as desired or could it be improved? The flow chart can be used as the basis for decision making and increased precision in the flow of patients through the same day surgery process.

A histogram is used to measure how frequently something occurs. A particular application of a histogram is reflected in the pareto chart of emergency department admissions shown in Figure 10-7. Pareto charts are among the most commonly used graphic displays for data. The pareto chart is used to determine frequency and priori-

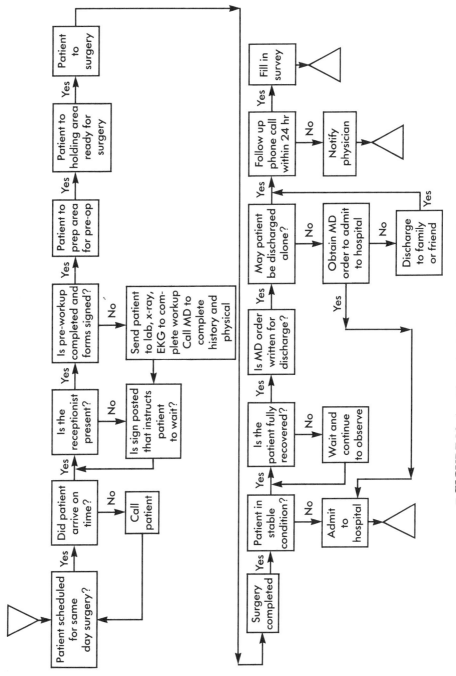

■ FIGURE 10-6   Flow chart of process of same day surgery.

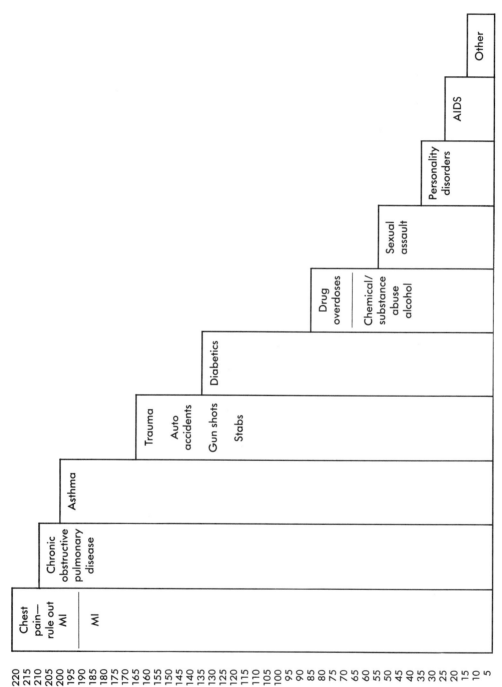

■ **FIGURE 10-7** Pareto chart of emergency department admissions.

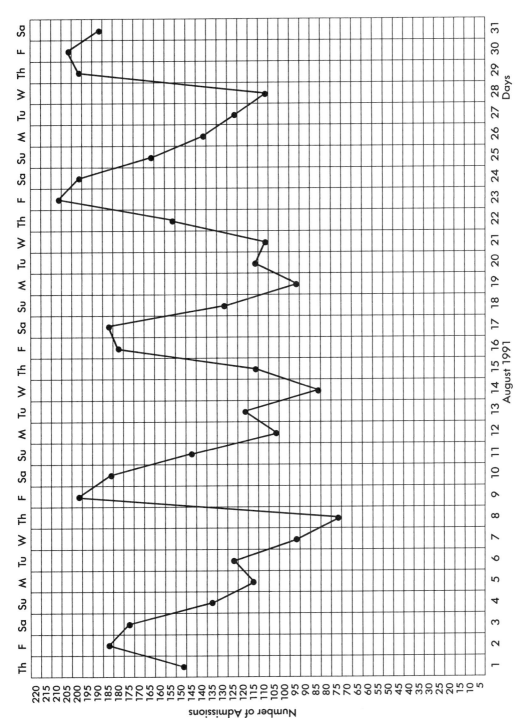

■ **FIGURE 10-8** Run chart of emergency department admissions per 24 hours.

ties. In the example shown in Figure 10-7, data were collected concerning all admissions to an emergency department. The bar farthest to the left represents the most frequent admissions and the bar farthest to the right represents the least frequent admissions. The pareto chart was used as a visual display of the most frequent to the least frequent number of admissions. This type of chart may assist in depicting the important aspects of care and service for a department as well as priorities for staff education.

A run chart is one of the simplest of the SPC tools. A run chart is used to document frequency over a period of time to illustrate trends. The example in Figure 10-8 tracks data for the number of emergency department admissions for the month of August 1991. It is evident that admissions peak on the weekends. This chart would support increased staffing during the most busy hours in the emergency department.

Possibly the most popular SPC tool is the control chart, which Dr. Deming often talks about as necessary to analyze processes. The purpose of the control chart, he emphasizes, is "to stop people from chasing down causes."[7] Properly understood and used, a control chart is a continuing guide to constant improvement. In addition, control charts are easy to use.

A control chart is simply a run chart with statistically determined upper and lower limits drawn on either side of the process average. The upper and lower control limits are determined by allowing a process to run as usual, without tampering and then analyzing the results. Every process has some variation. The more finely tuned the process, the less deviation there is from the average. Figure 10-1 is an example of a simple control chart. The threshold parameter forms shown in Figures 10-3 and 10-4 incorporate control charts.

■ WHO SHOULD EVALUATE THE VARIATIONS?

Once a variation requiring investigation is identified, it should be evaluated by those directly involved in the aspect of care to be examined. The traditional approach in health care has been to have the work of clinical staff evaluated by a QA coordinator. This QA coordinator functioned like a police officer.

Eskildson and Yates state that "This policing environment encourages data-collection delays and roadblocks, game playing, and conflict between . . . departments and QA over methods of data collection and analysis and over conclusions."[3] Fast feedback is essential to effective quality improvement; the lack of teamwork and the separation of "duties" has tended to erect barriers to speedy data collection and analysis. These barriers delay identification of the causes of the problem. Fast feedback requires that those who collect the data also do the analysis.

Separation of these tasks not only impedes quality management, it undermines teamwork, delays feedback and progress, increases costs of data gathering, and communicates a less than total organizational commitment to quality.[3]

THE BLUEPRINT council structure (see Chapter 4) recommends a central quality management council with membership drawn from every nursing department and ancillary department within the organization. This council is the governing, *authoritative* body for quality management within the organization. It coordinates quality management studies and functions as the central clearinghouse for all quality data and analysis within the organization.

Those delivering the care are involved in its monitoring and evaluation. The analysis of variations found during the studies is performed by the person(s) or group collecting the data. This analysis is then submitted to the quality management council.

■ HOW TO ANALYZE THE VARIATION

Once the data have been collected and organized, the variance decision-making tree presented in Figure 10-9 can be used to analyze the variation. To begin the study analysis, staff should ask, "Do the monitoring results fall outside the established threshold parameters?" If the answer is "no" and if no pattern or trend is apparent, then no corrective action is necessary and the monitoring schedule should be continued. If however, the answer to the question is "yes," the specific domain(s) involved in causing the variation must be identified. If patient variables are the cause of the variation, a clinical action plan is necessary. This may be in the form of a practice guideline, critical path, patient teaching plan, and the like. If patient variables are not the cause, staff or system variables are looked to as a source of the variation. (Patient, staff, and system variables were defined in step 4 and are listed on the indicator

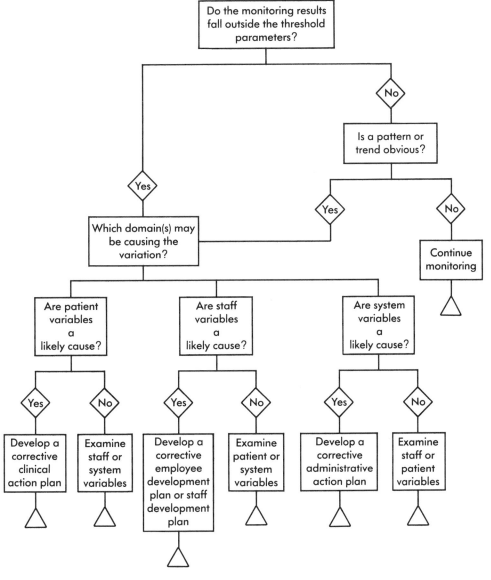

■ FIGURE 10-9   Variance decision-making tree.

development form described in Chapter 7.) Next the determination is made concerning whether staff variables were responsible for the variance. If so, the development and implementation of an employee development plan and/or staff development plan are indicated. If staff variables are not the cause of the variance, system or patient variables are looked to as causative factors. Finally it is questioned whether system variables are responsible for the variation in monitoring results. If they are, an administrative action plan is needed to correct the variance and bring the system into control. If they are not, patient and staff variables are looked to as causative factors.

In some cases, two or all three of the domains may contribute to the variance and multiple plans may be necessary to correct the deviation. It may also be necessary to review the indicator development form and reexamine the patient, staff, and system variables, adding additional sources of variance if the initial ones are not sufficient to fully explain the variation in results. In Chapter 11, the types of action planning required in each domain to correct the problem variables are described in detail.

If the answer to the question, "Do the monitoring results fall outside of the established threshold parameters?" is no, the next question becomes, "Is a trend or pattern in monitoring results obvious?" The threshold parameter form is reviewed to note any trends in monitoring results. If the answer to this question is no, the variation is probably common cause and the system is probably in statistical control with a variation due to chance. Because corrective action might result in tampering, it is probably best to wait until the next monitoring period and compare the results to see if a trend is forming. If, however, a trend or pattern does exist, this may indicate a special cause variation, which requires analysis of the patient, staff, and/or system variables that are causing the variance and the initiation of appropriate action planning.

The variance decision-making tree creates a trifocus for problem solving that helps to isolate the likely causes of variation in monitoring results. The more quickly sources of problems can be pinpointed, the more quickly solutions can be designed and implemented. Swift solutions to problems result in cost savings and improved patient care.

Rafael Aguayo says, "The companies that rely on inspection to improve quality believe that quality is expensive (because of the way they believe improvements are made). The Deming companies, on the other hand, are constantly improving the process and the product without justifying every improvement, confident that higher productivity, lower costs, and higher profits will result."[1]

"Ignorance is the most expensive commodity in the world."[1] In today's health care environment, nurses can no longer ignore the resource-saving, cost-effective statistical methods of monitoring and evaluating the care they provide.

REFERENCES

1. Aguayo R: Dr. Deming: the American who taught the Japanese about quality, New York, 1990, Carol Publishing Co.
2. Deming WE: Out of the crisis, Cambridge, Mass, 1986, Massachusetts Institute of Technology Center for Advanced Engineering Study.
3. Eskildson L and Yates GR: Lessons from industry: reusing organizational structure to improve health care quality assurance, Quality Rev Bull 17(2):38-41, 1991.
4. Ishikawa K: Guide to quality control, Tokyo, 1982, Asian Productivity Organization.
5. New nursing standards thrust hospitals into QI, Hospital Peer Rev, pp 136-138, Sept 1990.
6. O'Leary D: President's column, Joint Commission Perspective 10:2, Nov/Dec 1990.
7. Scholtes PR: The team handbook, Madison, Wis, 1990, Joiner Associates.
8. Sines B: Personal communication, April 21, 1991.
9. Walton M: Deming management method, New York, 1986, The Putnam Publishing Co.
10. Walton M: Deming management at work, New York, 1990, GP Putnam's Sons.

11

STEP 8:
TAKING ACTION

Those who fail to plan, plan to fail.
ANONYMOUS

It was a manufacturer's worst nightmare come true. On September 29, 1982, the first of seven Chicagoans died after ingesting cyanide-laced Extra Strength Tylenol capsules. This incident panicked the public and rocked the very foundation of Johnson & Johnson, the parent company of McNeil Laboratories, the maker of Tylenol.

Something needed to be done and quickly. However, the wrong move could worsen rather than correct the problem. Within hours of the incident, the switchboards at Johnson & Johnson were overloaded with calls from pharmacies, doctors, hospitals, poison control centers, and consumers, not to mention news reporters.

Recognizing the need for swift and decisive action, Johnson & Johnson executives mobilized a three-phase plan of action. Phase one involved problem identification and containment. By the end of the first day, the executives were convinced the poisonings did not originate at the plant, either accidentally or intentionally. This was confirmed the next morning, when the capsules taken by the sixth victim were identified to have been from a lot that had been produced at another location. Containment required the recall of all Tylenol capsules—over 31 million packages nationwide. The company also halted all further production of the capsules and suspended advertising of the product.

The second phase involved communication between the company, the police, the health authorities, and the public. Clarification of the incident was made in advertisements, letters to the trade, and statements to the media. Emergency phone lines were installed to answer questions.

By the second weekend, the company had moved into the third phase: rebuilding the brand name. (The idea of ending all further production of Tylenol was never a consideration, although industry experts suggested reintroducing the product under a new name.) The rebuilding phase involved a strategic plan that included reestablishing public trust in the product. A triple-seal, tamper-resistant package was designed. Coupons were distributed to the public offering free packages of Tylenol, and higher than normal discounts were given to retailers so that shelf space for Tylenol would be regained. Johnson & Johnson offered a $100,000 reward to anyone who provided information leading to the arrest and conviction of those responsible for the tragedy.

As a result of this incident, the Food and Drug Administration (FDA) and the over-the-counter pharmaceuticals organization formed a committee to develop standards for tamper-resistant packages. Previously, Tylenol had commanded about 35% of the $1.3 billion analgesic market, outselling the next four leading analgesics combined, but during the crisis, sales of Tylenol dropped 80%. By February 1983, however, Tylenol had regained almost 70% of its former market share.

The tragedy could have meant the end of Tylenol production and a significant blow to Johnson & Johnson. Success was achieved because swift and decisive action was taken.[1,6,10]

The story illustrates a critical point. To solve problems effectively or seize opportunities for quality improvement, a plan is necessary. The key to effective action is to act not to react. Successful action requires a strategy. "Strategy is not about adaptability in behavior, but about regularity, not about discontinuity but about consistency. Organizations adopt strategies to reduce uncertainties, to set direction, focus effort, reduce risks, and define the organization."[3]

Step 8 of the ten-step process requires proactive quality improvement. In the previous steps, efforts were geared to identifying the major service areas for which quality is paramount (quality awareness) and validating the achievement of predetermined levels of quality within these areas (quality appraisal). This step initiates the quality improvement phase of the process.

■ WHAT IS QUALITY IMPROVEMENT?

Quality improvement involves the resolution of quality problems and the exploitation of quality opportunities. Quality problems are either unsatisfactory or undesired patient outcomes or those obstacles within the service that interfere with achievement of desired patient outcomes. These problems may be clinical, professional, or administrative in nature. A clinical quality problem might be an increase in the number of injury-related falls. A professional quality problem might be a deficit in documentation of nursing process. An administrative quality problem might be inadequate staffing to meet patients' needs during the night.

Quality opportunities consist of those occasions when, although the quality threshold is adequate, an opportunity exists to improve the outcome of the service or the process by which the service is delivered. These situations provide the opportunity to "work smarter," not harder, to add value to the service while controlling costs. They may be clinical, professional, or administrative. For example, although the surgical wound infection rate falls to within the desired threshold parameter, staff may identify an opportunity to decrease costs without compromising patient outcomes by replacing sterile dressings with clean ones in dressing changes. Thus, while the threshold parameter is maintained, cost of service may be considerably reduced.

Inherent in quality improvement is change. In 500 BC Heraclitus said that nothing endures but change. More recently, both Waterman[12] and Peters[11] have discussed change as a necessary factor in today's corporate environment. Waterman defines change as a dynamic imbalance. "There is a kind of rhythm to the process: first, a constant search for standard ways of doing things that makes life easier. Then, the deliberate breaking of old rules, familiar patterns, past practice. . . ."[12]

Change is indicated whenever there is a discrepancy between what is actual and what is desired. The discrepancy can involve either the outcomes, the process, or the structure of the service. Improvements in the nosocomial infection rate or in patient compliance are examples of a change in desired clinical outcomes. A change in practice patterns such as the discontinuation of bedside-based laboratory monitoring is an example of a process change. A structure change might involve expanding the level of personnel who can perform certain clinical procedures.

Change is a complex, continuous process. Brooten describes it as a process that leads to alterations in individual or institutional patterns of behavior.[2] It may occur haphazardly or in an organized manner. Haphazard change simply happens. Brooten calls it "change by drift" and suggests that it is caused by benign neglect. It is marked by failure to consider the consequences of a series of actions. The spiralling costs of health care are an example of this type of change. The parties involved are carried along by the change much like a boat adrift in a sea. The process is undirected and the results are unpredictable.

A second type of change is reactive change. Spurred by an unmanageable situation (the proverbial straw that broke the camel's back) what happens can be described as a "knee jerk" reaction. For example, the mother of the chairman of the board received cold meals during a recent hospital stay. Memos and directives are issued and policies and procedures are immediately changed. Reactive change can have positive or negative results; however, the greatest problem with this type of change is that it is situational.

Planned change, on the other hand, is a deliberate, conscious, controlled process. It is proactive, involving collaborative goal setting and active participation by the parties involved. Activity is directed toward achievement of predefined outcomes.

Change requires movement. In haphazard change, the movement is uncontrolled. Reactive change is controlled, but the results may not be optimal because of lack of forethought. During planned change, there is a deliberate attempt to control the change process by predetermining outcomes and adjusting the operating systems to achieve the desired results.

■ PLANNING FOR CHANGE

Planned change necessitates a strategy for change. Resolution of quality problems or exploitation of quality opportunities requires strategic planning.

Strategic planning is the vehicle for responding to and shaping change by developing and implementing outcome-directed strategies to manage that change. "Strategic planning is a continuous, systematic process of making risk-taking decisions today with the greatest knowledge of their effects on the future; organizing efforts necessary to carry out these decisions; and evaluating results of those decisions against expected outcomes through reliable feedback mechanisms."[5] It is the process of making decisions about the design and delivery of the important aspects of clinical, professional, and administrative services. Strategic planning turns desired results into a plan of action.

■ IS PLANNING NECESSARY?

In the midst of constant change, planning provides stability. In today's health care economy, organizations *cannot* afford *not* to plan. Garner suggests, however, that the same factors that necessitate planning are also the acknowledged reasons given for not planning.[7] These pressures include service diversification, competition, changing consumer preferences, accelerated technology, economic constraints, changing professional expectations, and organizational complexity.

The benefits of planning are numerous. Planning establishes standards by which performance can be evaluated. It provides a sense of direction. It determines limits by building in controls that focus full attention on the task at hand. It assigns responsibility and accountability for process and outcomes. A strategic plan provides a barometer to measure variance from the intended path while affording an organized approach to complex projects or problems. It reduces the costs of human and material resources by focusing on their effective and efficient use. It is a lifesaver when crisis strikes because it provides the necessary redirection in the midst of chaos. Had Johnson & Johnson failed to plan, Tylenol may have been lost forever.

Planning facilitates collaboration and creativity because it focuses on a critical issue and fosters the exchange and development of new ideas and solutions. Planning, however, is a skill in which many individuals lack expertise. This may account for some reluctance to plan. Other reasons for not planning relate to the problems inherent in the traditional approach to strategic planning.

■ REDEFINING THE STRATEGIC PLAN

The traditional strategic plan set the overall goals and direction for the organization. It was global in scope, dealing with ways to maximize market position and financial outcomes. It was generally considered to be an executive function and often remained exclusively in the board room. The focus was projecting a 5-year plan to move the institution toward its vision.

Today's organizational visions are much shorter ranging since the economic and technologic stability of health care is constantly changing. Thus, the entire approach to strategic planning needs to be rethought. Today's plans need to focus on the short term. One-year plans now replace the replanning syndrome of the past wherein much time was spent generating 3- to 5-year plans that had to be redesigned within a year because of unpredicted change. This also contributed to a reluctance to participate in the planning process and reinforced the perception of planning as an academic exercise.

No longer is planning an executive function. Today strategic planning is an essential tool for the entire organization. It is a critical element whenever and wherever change is needed at the divisional, unit, or individual level. Committees and task forces also need to use strategic planning to manage change. Garner suggests "Not only do health care organizations need a vibrant and results oriented planning process but planning is crucial at all organizational levels."[7] The 3M Company develops a new strategic plan each year. Each of its businesses outlines its strategy for the year and submits it to headquarters, where a corporate plan is developed.

The traditional view of strategic planning is changing. Peters suggests that flexibility in planning is the watchword of the future.[11] The planning process and therefore, the plan itself is dynamic. To be responsive, flexible, and customer-driven, the process must be "bottom-up," i.e., it must start at the front line and include those staff members who will implement the change. Decisions regarding the plan must be made by those parties expected to carry out the plan.

■ DECISIONS, DECISIONS, DECISIONS

Decision making is a critical skill in the planning process. Unlike routine or operational decision making, which focuses on day-to-day situations, strategic decision making involves new ways to do things or to solve problems on a large scale. Decisions are made in all three phases of planning.

In the first phase, priority setting, decisions are made regarding which critical issues will be addressed and whether those issues are clinical, professional, or administrative in nature. Decisions are also made regarding priorities for action based on which issues have the greatest influence on patient outcomes. The important aspects of the care/service grid (Chapter 6) are helpful in making these decisions.

In the next phase, outcome setting, decision making focuses on the results to be achieved for each of the defined priorities. Questions to be asked include "What are the desired outcomes for this critical issue?" and "What will the results of this planned change in service be?" If, for example, the critical issue is documentation, the desired outcomes of a quality documentation system must be defined before any attempt is made to change the current system. One outcome might be that there will be a legally sound record of nursing activities and patient responses to those activities. Another might be the elimination of redundancy or a decrease in charting time. This is the phase that clearly separates planned change from reactive change.

Many organizations omit this phase of the planning process. They plan activities, implement them, and wait to see the results. Determining outcomes is critical to ensuring that the planned activities focus on achieving desired results. No resources are wasted on extraneous or nonessential, nonproductive activities. All actions are directed and purposeful.

The third phase, intervention planning, involves deciding how to achieve the predetermined outcomes. Decisions include who will do what by when. Outlining "who" will act delegates the responsibility, awards the authority, and establishes accountability for completing specific activities. The "what" or specified activities must include only those actions essential to accomplish the desired results. Actions must be resource driven and sequential. Being resource driven means that the constraints of people, equipment, operating systems, money, and other resources are considered when making activity choices. The "by when" portion of this phase defines the completion date for specific activities. It provides a time line to ensure achieving the outcome by the target date.

■ DEVELOPING AN EFFECTIVE PLAN

Curtin states "the most successful strategies for action or change capitalize on existing value structures."[3] These value structures are evident in written standards. The box below lists the policies that must be in effect for successful planning. These policies or rules for plans must be adhered to diligently.

Deep and Sussman describe four inhibitions that prevent good planning.[4] The first is that many people consider planning a luxury. They are so busy "putting out

---

POLICIES FOR PLANS

1. Plans must be written.
2. Plans must be developed with input from staff responsible for implementation.
3. Plans must be specific to the defined critical issue.
4. Plans must be realistic.
5. Plans must be flexible.
6. Plans must define outcomes, actions, and responsible parties.
7. Plans must be reviewed and/or revised periodically.
8. People affected by the plan must be kept informed.
9. Planned actions and outcomes must be timed.
10. The timespan of a plan must be no longer than 1 year.

ELEVEN CHARACTERISTICS OF AN EFFECTIVE PLAN

These features must all be in place before the plan is implemented:

1. It is stated clearly in terms of the desired end results.
2. It is put into writing.
3. It has been drafted by people who will also be responsible for its implementation.
4. It has been communicated to all those it affects for their comments.
5. One person is ultimately accountable for its implementation.
6. A specific date is established for its completion; earlier dates are established for intermediate milestones as appropriate.
7. Criteria for success of the plan and how to apply those criteria are determined.
8. Intermediate review steps for "go/no go" decisions or revisions of the plan are laced throughout the implementation period.
9. Potential problems that may arise during implementation are identified and anticipated with preventive action.
10. Potential opportunities that may arise during implementation are identified so as to take advantage of them.
11. The supervisor of the plan is held accountable for reporting progress and revisions to the plan on a regular basis to superiors and to all those involved with implementation.

From Deep S and Sussman L: Smart moves, © 1990, Addison-Wesley Publishing Co, Inc, Reading, Mass. Used with permission.

fires" that they cannot free themselves from their immediate activities to focus on tomorrow. Second, because planning is a future-oriented activity, many feel that it constitutes little more than an educated guess. A third obstacle is society's emphasis on doing rather than thinking. "We erect statues and name streets after people who successfully execute the plan, not those who devise it."[4] Finally, Deep and Sussman believe that many people lack planning skills. They suggest that firefighters, uncertainty avoiders, doers, and skill-deficient individuals can benefit from simple, straightforward planning advice. They offer the 11 characteristics of an effective plan listed in the box above.

■ WRITING EFFECTIVE OUTCOMES

Probably the most difficult part of planning for most health care professionals is writing outcomes. This may be because they are accustomed to carrying out actions and waiting to see the results. In the implementation phase, this is exactly what happens. However, in the planning phase, the desired outcomes must be devised *first*, then the activities required to achieve those outcomes must be designed. It is only after the action plan has been developed that the implementation phase begins. It is during this phase that the planned activities are carried out and it is noted whether these activities produce the desired results. Figure 11-1 depicts the relationship of process and outcome during planning and implementation.

Without well-written outcomes, the planning process is doomed to fail. Outcomes provide the foundation for all actions that follow. They represent the difference between motion and direction. Without them, activities have no focus. The effective planner writes SMART outcomes:

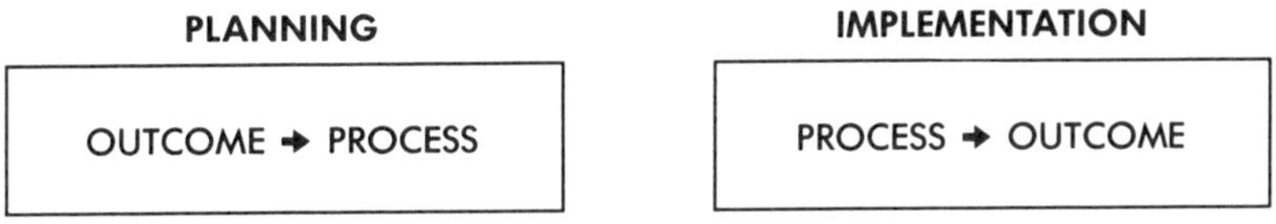

PLANNING

IMPLEMENTATION

OUTCOME ➝ PROCESS

PROCESS ➝ OUTCOME

■ FIGURE 11-1   Relationship of process and outcome during planning and implementation.

Responsible party	Who	5 West staff
Outcome verb	Will Do	will increase
Conditions	What	their compliance to the alteration in skin integrity protocol
Criteria	By how much, When	by 10% in one year

■ FIGURE 11-2   Anatomy of an outcome.

Specific:	Define only one intention/result per outcome.
Measurable:	Quantify the intention/result.
Appropriate:	Ensure the intention/result is suitable for the identified critical issue.
Realistic:	Set challenging but achievable results given the available resources.
Timed:	State when the result is to be achieved.

Outcomes must be written in terms of the results to be achieved—not how to get there. For example, "The staff will reduce the number of level IV falls in geriatric patients to less than 5% within 6 months" rather than "The staff will develop a falls prevention program." The first is a result, the second is an action designed to achieve the result. To facilitate this process, use results-oriented verbs such as increase, decrease, reduce, maintain, expand, eliminate, improve; rather than process verbs such as design, develop, identify, evaluate.

An effective outcome defines who will do what by how much, when. Figure 11-2 depicts the anatomy of an outcome. Depending on the type of plan needed, outcomes may be clinical, professional, or administrative in nature.

■ DEVELOPING CLINICAL PLANS

When the critical issue for change deals with patient care, the written plan is a clinical one. In the first phase of clinical planning, the critical issue to be decided is the type of clinical plan to be used. Clinical action plans include standardized care plans, critical paths, discharge plans, protocols/practice guidelines, and patient teaching plans. Depending on the clinical situation and the nursing care delivery system, the type of plan utilized may vary. Nevertheless, in a resource-driven environment, decisions must be made regarding appropriate priorities of care relative to the patient's

■

JOINT COMMISSION'S 1992 NURSING STANDARDS

NC.1.3.4   The patient's medical record includes documentation of
  NC.1.3.4.1   the initial assessments and reassessments;
  NC.1.3.4.2   the nursing diagnoses and/or patient care needs;
  NC.1.3.4.3   the interventions identified to meet the patient's nursing care needs;
  NC.1.3.4.4   the nursing care provided;
  NC.1.3.4.5   the patient's response to, and the outcomes of, the care provided; and
  NC.1.3.4.6   the abilities of the patient and/or, as appropriate, his/her significant other(s) to manage continuing care needs after discharge.
NC.1.3.5   Nursing care data related to patient assessments, the nursing care planned, nursing interventions, and patient outcomes are permanently integrated into the clinical information system (for example, the medical record).

From Joint Commission on Accreditation of Health Care Organizations: Nursing care, Accreditation manual for hospitals, Chicago, 1992, JCAHO.

phase of acuity, projected length of stay, and available resources. For example, given a length of stay of 3.5 days for a mastectomy patient, resolution of body image disturbance is not a realistic outcome. A more appropriate result might be that the patient is able to use existing coping mechanisms to manage the emotional trauma associated with breast removal.

The decisions in the second phase relate to defining patient outcomes. Patient outcomes may be desired or expected. Desired outcomes are those results you wish to obtain as a result of specific nursing interventions. Expected outcomes are those you can anticipate as a result of medical or nursing intervention. For example, fever, nausea, and vomiting are expected outcomes of chemotherapy. The desired outcome in this situation might be that the patient maintains his or her current weight during the treatment period or that the patient's fluid and electrolyte balance is maintained within plus or minus 10% during the treatment period. Certain things happen as a result of medical and nursing therapy; it is important to recognize these expected results and take them into consideration when writing outcomes. Controlling the fever, nausea, and vomiting is a means to an end. These activities are necessary to achieve the desired results whether the results are maintaining weight, fluid and electrolyte balance, or comfort.

Clinical outcomes are patient focused, not nurse focused. For example, "The patient's fluid and electrolyte balance will be maintained within plus or minus 10% during the treatment period" rather than "The nurse will monitor the patient's fluid and electrolytes."

In the third phase of clinical planning, the decisions revolve around which activities are essential to assist the patient in achieving the predetermined outcomes. Those activities may be referred to as interventions or orders. "Successful nursing orders depend upon the nurse's ability to generate and choose alternatives that will most likely be effective."[8] Interventions are delineated for each of the defined patient outcomes. Each of the actions then identifies who will do what by when. The "who" may be the nurse, another health care worker, the patient, or a significant other. While the outcomes are patient centered, the activities carried out to achieve those outcomes may be performed by any number of individuals. It is up to the nurse to determine who is best suited to complete the tasks. The "what" defines the action or task to be performed and the "when" defines the deadline for completion.

The use of traditional nursing care plans has recently become a controversial topic especially since the 1992 Joint Commission standards have eliminated any direct reference to their use. Some have interpreted the elimination of a standard requiring evidence of a care plan on the patient's chart to mean that it is no longer necessary to plan care. This is not so. The Joint Commission's nursing standard N.C.1.3.4 and its substandards and N.C.1.3.5 clearly define the need to utilize the nursing process in documenting care.[9] These standards appear in the box on page 166.

■ DEVELOPING A PROFESSIONAL PRACTICE PLAN

When the quality issue to be addressed involves the staff who provide the service, the improvement plan must focus on the practitioner. Two types of plans are commonly used: the employee development plan and the staff development plan.

The Employee Development Plan

The employee development plan is used when a staff performance problem occurs or when there is an opportunity to facilitate the growth and development of an individual. In the first phase of planning for performance correction the nature of the performance problem must be determined. Figure 11-3 depicts a performance prob-

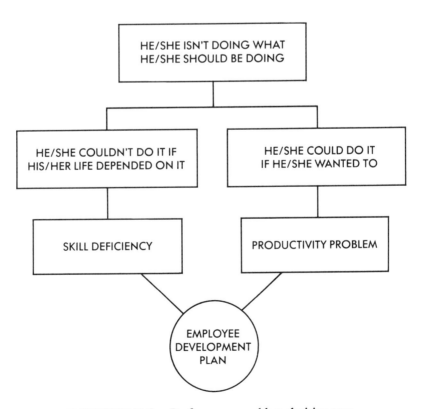

■ FIGURE 11-3   Performance problem decision tree.

EMPLOYEE'S NAME _____

DATE OF PLAN _____

Area for Development	Expected Outcome	Target Date/ Monitor(s)	Actions	Responsible Persons	Completion Date		Incentive
					Projected	Actual	

Employee Signature _____ Date _____

Nurse Manager _____ Date _____

■ FIGURE 11-4 Employee development plan.

lem decision tree. The problem may relate to competency or productivity, the two components of performance. Competency is the ability to do something at some level of proficiency. It is composed of some combination of knowledge, skills, attitudes, and values. Productivity is the application of knowledge, skills, attitudes, or values to yield favorable or useful results.

An employee development plan can be helpful regardless of the nature of the performance problem. Achieving an individual's potential is also facilitated by the use of this plan. In the first phase, the critical areas for development or improvement are identified. In the second phase, outcomes are defined for each critical issue. These outcomes focus on the individual staff member, and define the results necessary to demonstrate an improvement in performance or an achievement of potential. Next, activities necessary to fulfill the outcomes are specified. A sample format for an employee development plan is shown in Figure 11-4. The benefits of an employee development plan include:

- It increases staff control over their own practice through a self-administered improvement plan.
- It increases staff accountability for their own performance.
- It shifts focus of control from a conventional manager-imposed system to self-control.
- It provides staff with a personal barometer against which to measure growth.

The employee development plan is self-directed and self-administered. The employee, with the assistance of the nurse manager, develops the plan. Together they identify critical elements for development or improvement. Then, outcomes are determined and specific activities outlined with a time line for each element. The employee and the nurse manager negotiate an incentive package for successful plan completion. The employee then implements the plan and periodically reviews and documents progress with the nurse manager, who acts as a facilitator in this process. In a peer review system, the staff nurse employee would present documentation of successful completion to the peer review body who would then decide upon promotion.

The Staff Development Plan

When there is a competency deficit in more than one staff member or when an opportunity exists to expand the potential of more than one individual, the staff development plan is used. Issues that require a staff development plan might include preparation of staff to implement nursing diagnosis, or the development of computer literacy skills. Another example might be a plan to certify all the critical care nurses in advanced life support or as CCRNs. The process of planning is similar to that used for the employee development plan. A sample format for a staff development plan is shown in Figure 11-5.

The benefits of staff development planning include:

- Timely and appropriate education of staff
- Establishment of a link between quality assurance and staff development
- Improved consistency in educational planning

The education department is responsible for the development, implementation, and evaluation of the staff development plan. These three areas of responsibility may be

Critical Issue	Learner Objectives	Learning Activities	Responsible Person(s)	Completion Date		Evaluation Methodology	Threshold		Remarks
				Projected	Actual		Projected	Actual	

■ FIGURE 11-5 Staff development plan.

carried out solely by the education department or in conjunction with other clinical or managerial staff within the division of nursing.

■ DEVELOPING AN ADMINISTRATIVE ACTION PLAN

In the administrative domain, an administrative action plan is the tool of choice. It is used when a quality problem or opportunity related to the system is to be addressed. Examples of administrative issues include implementation of a new system, e.g., patient classification, care delivery, use of a new subcontractor for laboratory services; a merger or acquisition; reorganization of the organization or division; and development of a yearly performance plan. Any time systems must change, an administrative action plan is needed. In the first phase of planning, decision making focuses on which priorities must be addressed first. Being resource driven, priority is given to those changes that will have the greatest effect on patient outcomes. In the second phase, outcomes are developed to specify the desired results of administrative change and its anticipated impact on the system. System outcomes deal with ways in which the organization must change to effect quality care. Reducing overtime hours as a percentage of total hours worked is one example of a system outcome. Another might involve reducing the salary cost per patient day, or reducing the absentee rate. Finally, specific actions are outlined that will facilitate the achievement of the defined outcomes. Figure 11-6 provides a sample format for an administrative action plan.

Administrative action planning may be used by many groups or individuals. For example, the ENC develops a strategic plan, the QMC develops the monitoring and evaluation plan, and a task force may develop a plan to implement primary nursing. A nurse manager uses the administrative action plan to outline the achievement of annual department objectives, and the quality management coordinator may use an administrative action plan to computerize the data collection and analysis system.

The benefits of administrative action planning are numerous. They include:

- The integration of service at all levels within the department or organization
- Coordination of managerial activities
- Improved utilization of resources

These benefits are realized because the process of planning focuses attention on the individuals or groups involved in and affected by a change and the resources necessary to effect that change. The mere act of planning means that attention is given to what results are needed and what is the most efficient way of obtaining those results. Managerial responsibilities then revolve around providing the environment in which those planned activities can happen.

Following the example of previous chapters for pain management in terminally ill cancer patients, analysis of the variance may lead to the development of a number of different plans. A patient teaching plan might be indicated if analysis reveals that patients are uncomfortable because they are not using the equipment correctly. An employee development plan might be indicated if a particular staff nurse is having difficulty passing the credentialing examination. A staff development plan may be designed if analysis indicates an overall need for nurses to reassess their values related to pain management. Finally, an administrative action plan and budget modifications may be needed if analysis of variance defines the lack of patient-controlled analgesia units to be a factor in achieving satisfactory levels of pain control in terminally ill cancer patients.

Critical Issue	Desired Outcome	Target Date	Actions	Completion Date		Responsible Person(s)
				Projected	Actual	

■ FIGURE 11-6   Department of nursing administrative action plan.

■ TURNING PLANS INTO ACTION

It is not enough to create good plans; they must be enacted. A plan is no better than the paper on which it is written if it is not implemented. Without action, the plan is simply rhetorical, a statement of intended performance. The proof is in the pudding.

Moving the plan from paper to practice is facilitated by establishing timetables for completion of specific activities and assigning responsibility for accomplishment of those tasks. Each responsible party must act in accordance with the plan and complete the assigned activities in the time allotted, if the plan is to succeed.

The key to successful action is planning. The traditional view of planning must change from that of an academic exercise to that of a dynamic tool used at every level of the organization.

Decision making is the heart of planning and occurs in each of the three phases of the process. In the initial phase of planning, the decisions relate to identification of the critical issues and establishment of priorities for action. In the second phase, decision making centers on the desired outcomes to be achieved, and in the final phase, decisions are made regarding the actions needed to accomplish the outcomes.

Plans take many forms and may address clinical, professional, or administrative priorities. Regardless of the type of plan, however, as one anonymous sage put it, one must

> Plan purposefully
> Prepare prayerfully
> Proceed positively
> and
> Pursue persistently.

REFERENCES

1. A death blow for Tylenol? Business Week, p 151, Oct 18, 1982.
2. Brooten D, Hayman L, and Naylor M: Leadership for change, ed 2, Philadelphia, 1988, JB Lippincott.
3. Curtin L: Creating a culture of competence, Nurs Manage 21(9):7-8, 1990.
4. Deep S and Sussman L: Smart moves, Reading, Mass, 1990, Addison-Wesley.
5. Drucker P: Management: tasks, responsibilities, policies, New York, 1974, Harper & Row Publishers.
6. Fannin R: Diary of an amazing comeback, Market Media Decis, special ed, pp 129-133, Spring 1982.
7. Garner J, Smith H, and Piland N: Strategic nursing management, Rockville, 1990, Aspen Publishers.
8. Iyer P, Taptich B, and Bernocchi-Losey D: Nursing process and nursing diagnosis, Philadelphia, 1986, WB Saunders.
9. Joint Commission on Accreditation of Health Care Organizations: Nursing care. In Accreditation manual for hospitals, Chicago, 1992, JCAHO.
10. Moore T: The fight to save Tylenol, Fortune, pp 45-49, Nov 29, 1982.
11. Peters T: Thriving on chaos, New York, 1988, Knopf.
12. Waterman RH Jr: The renewal factor, New York, 1987, Bantam Books.

12

STEP 9:
ASSESSING ACTIONS AND
DOCUMENTING IMPROVEMENT

Process is not necessarily progress.
JACKIE KATZ

Perhaps you have heard the story about the patient who went to see his psychiatrist, wearing only a fireman's hat. His entire body was painted purple with red polka dots. He was flapping his arms wildly and clucking like a chicken while he hopped on one foot and then the other. When his doctor asked him what he thought he was doing, the man replied, "I'm keeping the elephants away!" "But we're in the middle of Manhattan," stated the psychiatrist, "there aren't any elephants here." "See how good it works!" exclaimed the patient with a smile.

The ninth step of the Joint Commission's monitoring and evaluation process is designed to see "how good it works." As with the patient's plan above, quality improvement plans may involve elaborate activities and also may consume valuable resources, but a flurry of activity does not guarantee the desired results. As with the staff nurse who at the end of a hectic day wonders exactly what has been accomplished, a plan can generate much work with little measurable return. The key to ensuring that the specific actions outlined in a plan are producing what they were intended to produce is periodic review and ongoing documentation of achievement.

This chapter focuses on the process of evaluating and documenting how the implementation of action plans designed in step 8 progressed. It discusses the differences between evaluative and diagnostic judgment, process versus outcome review, and quantitative versus qualitative analysis. It describes the followup necessary to validate and record the quality improvement that results from the activities outlined in the action plans.

All plans, whether they are clinical, professional, or administrative in nature, require followup analysis. This is the step in the process that provides documentation of not only the intent to act but the outcomes of that intent. In the absence of followup, data collection, analysis, and action planning are purely academic exercises. Followup evaluation is the grist from the mill of progress. It focuses on the action plan and analyzes both the ends and the means, the outcomes and the process, the results and the interventions. Too frequently, followup has focused only on the process of planning and whether or not the activities in the plan were carried out. Little, if any, attention was given to the results of the planned activities. The need to monitor the progress made toward the results for which the plan was designed and initiated is imperative.

Timing is everything in followup. Change takes time. If a change is evaluated too early, the expected results may not yet be apparent. A covert reason for a lack of quality improvement may be hasty remonitoring. Concurrent as well as retrospective review may help to eliminate this as a cause of less than optimal achievement. Concurrent review occurs while the plan is being carried out and focuses on the accomplishment of interim objectives. These interim objectives are benchmarks of progress along the way toward the ultimate desired outcomes. Retrospective review is carried out after all the interventions outlined in the plan have been completed.

Monitoring and evaluation does not end when actions are taken. Not only must staff continue to monitor the aspect of care for future opportunities for improvement, but to determine whether actions taken are successful in improving care or service. The results of continued monitoring and evaluation should provide information to make that determination.[3]

■ JUDGMENT: A CRITICAL DECISION-MAKING SKILL

Followup evaluation relies heavily on decision-making skills. Decision making requires judgment.

Bleich suggests that many experienced nurses are uncomfortable with taking responsibility for making and documenting judgments and therefore are reluctant to do so. Reasons for nurses' discomfort in making and documenting judgments might include lack of understanding, lack of skill, lack of consistent evaluative terminology, and accountability aversion.[1] One must understand what a judgment is and be skilled in making judgments so that there is confidence that the judgment is sound. Once a judgment is made and documented, the individual who made the judgment owns it and must be willing and able to defend it. The reluctance of professional nurses to make judgments is evidenced by the number of recommendations and contingencies cited by the Joint Commission in the area of documentation of the evaluation phase of the nursing process.

■ DIAGNOSTIC JUDGMENT

Bleich outlines two types of judgment—diagnostic and evaluative.[1] In general nurses tend to be more comfortable with the former.

Diagnostic judgment involves the collection, analysis, and synthesis of data. It is used during the assessment, diagnosis, and planning steps of the nursing process. There is a heavy emphasis on these steps in basic nursing education. Physical assessment, history taking, and formulating nursing diagnoses and care plans are stressed not only in basic nursing programs but also in continuing education conferences and seminars. The transition in the practice settings to the use of nursing diagnosis has necessitated increased proficiency in this area. Much time and effort has been spent, therefore, in improving nurses' skills in using their diagnostic judgment. Impetus for developing these skills has also come from the Joint Commission's nursing standards. Standard NC.1 states, "Patients receive nursing care based on a documented assessment of their needs." The standards continue to state that the assessment includes biophysical, psychosocial, environmental, self-care, educational, and discharge-planning factors based on identified nursing diagnosis and/or patient care needs.[3] Thus, the need for sophisticated skills in diagnostic judgment is well documented.

Diagnostic judgment focuses on problem identification, whether the problem is clinical, professional, or administrative. It can, however, also be used to identify opportunities for improvement where no problem currently exists. This is the preventive aspect of diagnostic judgment which enables nurses to identify potential problems or opportunities to intervene to improve the efficiency or the effectiveness of the process. Traditionally, the thrust of diagnostic judgment has been problem finding; consequently, nurses are less adept at using their diagnostic judgment for prevention. Problem finding may involve identifying the signs and symptoms of digoxin toxicity in a patient, identifying a lack of staff compliance with a new procedure, or the misappropriation of linen on the weekend shifts. Prevention, on the other hand, enables the nurse to identify symptoms of a potential problem, e.g., identifying patients at risk for digoxin toxicity, predicting staff's response to a new situation, or anticipating that the volume of linen required on a particular weekend will be heavier than usual.

To diagnose effectively, one must be able to synthesize. Synthesizing is having the ability to combine separate elements to form a coherent whole. For example, identifying that a patient's incision is red, painful, and warm to the touch, and that the sutures are taut, requires observation skills. To recognize that those symptoms may signal wound infection requires the ability to synthesize. "This is a process of working with elements, parts, etc. and combining them in such a way as to constitute a pattern or structure not clearly there before."[2] Combining collected data in ways that form patterns requires sophisticated analysis skills. Mapping trends in monitoring results is another example of synthesizing. For instance, data collection from six of eight departments may report a slight increase in the volume of injury-related falls in a specific quarter. Taken individually, each report may not be significant; however when viewed together, a major safety problem may be apparent. The preventive aspect of diagnostic judgment can also be seen in this example. Prevention of increases in injury-related falls may result from discovering and eliminating significant contributing factors such as heavily waxed floors or slippers with slick soles.

Using diagnostic judgment is like playing detective. It is the nurse's job to identify the various clues to a particular clinical, professional, or administrative problem and to determine the "culprit." Knowing the problem and the cause is only half the battle, however. Once the source of the problem is identified, the nurse uses his/her diagnostic judgment to devise a plan that will solve the problem once and for all.

In the previous steps of the ten-step process, diagnostic skills have been utilized. At this point however, a different kind of judgment is required.

▪ EVALUATIVE JUDGMENT

Evaluative judgment frustrates many nurses. Its absence is frequently cited in Joint Commission recommendations. Although many nurses confuse diagnostic and evaluative judgment, they are very different. Both require critical thinking skills, but diagnosis is not evaluation. Many nurses erroneously interchange the words "assessment" and "evaluation." These are two distinct processes, and, while assessment receives much attention in basic nursing education, evaluation frequently does not. Being able to differentiate the two is a critical first step in identifying when to use each.

Evaluation involves making judgments about the value of ideas, solutions, methods, or materials. It uses standards for appraising the extent to which actions or results are accurate, effective, economical, or satisfying. Evaluation can be quantitative or qualitative. An example of quantitative evaluation is the statement that the room temperature is 95° F as measured by thermometer. A qualitative corollary is "It's sweltering in here!" Quantitative evaluation involves numbers; qualitative evaluation involves perceptions.

According to Bloom, people evaluate, judge, or appraise almost everything they come in contact with. However, most of those judgments are highly egocentric, i.e., they are quick decisions made without much forethought and based on the individual's frame of reference. They fall more into the realm of opinion rather than judgment and into the unconscious rather than the conscious realm.[2] For example, if an owner is dissatisfied with the service on his or her car, that individual may choose never to purchase a car of that make again. While a rude or ineffective service representative may have had nothing to do with the quality of the car, an opinion is generalized about the company and its product based on a personal experience that may or may not reflect reality. Patients in hospitals may form similar opinions about the quality of the medical or nursing services based on their reactions to the "hotel" services they do or do not receive.

True evaluation, however, requires a conscious effort and is based on objective criteria.

Internal and External Criteria for Followup

Objective criteria are used to followup on the action plans formulated in the previous step. These criteria may be internal or external. Internal standards relate to the action plan itself. Is the plan consistent in approach? Is it on target? Internal standards are used to determine that there are no major errors in the format of the plan or the planning process, i.e., the plan design.

External standards relate to the appropriateness of the plan to achieve the desired ends. Did the plan produce the intended results? These criteria consider the efficiency, economy, or utility of specific activities to achieve specific results. Do the activities chosen represent the best solution to the problem posed? Are the activities chosen the most appropriate ones in light of the alternatives? Do the activities chosen produce results other than those desired?

In using the external standards, both the process and outcomes of the plan are analyzed. Process review is accomplished using formative evaluation, while outcome review requires the use of summative evaluation.

Formative Versus Summative Evaluation

Formative evaluations analyze the response to a specific intervention. Summative evaluations evaluate progress toward established outcomes. Formative evaluations look at the particular pieces of the action plan and the relative importance to the whole, while summative evaluations analyze how well (or how poorly) the pieces worked together to achieve the desired results. Formative evaluations therefore tend to focus on the process of carrying out the action plan and summative evaluations focus on the achievement or lack of achievement of outcomes.

Both formative and summative evaluations are used in the nursing process; the Joint Commission's ten-step monitoring and evaluation process. Figure 12-1 compares the use of diagnostic and evaluative judgments in both the nursing process and the monitoring and evaluation process. The dividing line between diagnostic and evaluative judgment is the implementation of the action plan. Whether that plan is a patient care plan, a teaching plan, an employee development plan, a staff development

Type of Judgment	Nursing Process Steps	Monitoring and Evaluation Activities
Diagnostic judgment	Assessment Diagnosis Planning	Data collection/analysis Problem/opportunity identification Action planning
Evaluative judgment	Evaluation	Evaluation of variation

■ FIGURE 12-1   Relationship of diagnostic and evaluative judgment and the nursing and monitoring and evaluation processes.

plan, or an administrative action plan, once the activities outlined in the plan are initiated, the type of critical thinking skills shifts from diagnostic to evaluative. Evaluative judgment analyzes the efficiency and effectiveness of the plan; therefore followup of the plan of action must include an efficiency and effectiveness analysis.

■ EVALUATING EFFICIENCY AND EFFECTIVENESS

Evaluation measures the overall efficiency and effectiveness of any set of activities designed to achieve a desired end. Efficiency is measured by process review. Outcome review measures effectiveness. Efficiency measures the relationship of what an organization gets out of the plan in comparison to what it puts into making the planned activities happen. Efficiency involves doing right things right. It requires working smarter, not harder.

Outcome evaluation deals with effectiveness. Effectiveness is the degree to which the activities outlined in the plan produced the desired results. Did the strategy work? Lancaster defines two major effectiveness criteria or standards. The first is appropriateness or accuracy, i.e., the fit between the problem or opportunity and the chosen strategy. The second criterion is resource allocation. Without proper allocation of resources, even the best strategy will fail.[4]

■ WHAT TO EVALUATE AND WHEN

First and foremost, the focus of the followup evaluation should be the effectiveness of the plan. Did the plan do what it was designed to do? Has the action plan achieved the desired results?

Evaluation of the effectiveness of the action plan is usually accomplished by remonitoring the original indicator. If, for example, a teaching plan was developed to teach terminally ill cancer patients how to use patient-controlled analgesia units, success or failure of the plan would be based on the increase in the patient's comfort level because of better understanding of how to use the equipment. Therefore, remonitoring the original aspect of care would indicate an improvement if the study results fell within the threshold parameters as a result of implementing the teaching plan when they did not fall within the parameters prior to patient teaching. By using the same study, the initial results can serve as a baseline to track the degree of progress or improvement.

There are three possible results that can be obtained by remonitoring the original study after action plan implementation:

1. *The desired results outlined in the plan were achieved.* The problem has been corrected or the opportunity capitalized upon. The predetermined outcomes have been achieved and the remonitoring data fall within the threshold parameters. In this case, the original monitoring and evaluation schedule is resumed to ensure that quality improvement is sustained.

2. *The desired results have not been met but there is significant progress toward their achievement.* Remonitoring data fall closer to the threshold parameters than the initial study. The problem seems to be resolving. In this case, a process review or formative evaluation is necessary in addition to the outcome review. In this review, the outcomes, actions, resources, and target dates are reevaluated and revised as necessary to facilitate the achievement of the desired results. Perhaps additional time is necessary to complete the activities because a crisis created a temporary diversion. Perhaps more resources are necessary to fully execute the plan. Perhaps some of the specified activities or interventions were out of sequence or were not carried out according to the timeline. Adjustment of the plan is necessary to meet the desired outcomes. Questions to ask during a process review include the following:

- Were the outcomes SMART (see Chapter 11)?
- Were the target dates for accomplishment realistic?
- Has enough time elapsed for the desired change to occur?
- Were the actions/interventions carried out as specified?
- Were sufficient resources allocated for the accomplishment of the results?

Once the plan has been revised, it must be implemented and evaluated by remonitoring the original indicator once again to see if the changes have produced the necessary improvement to boost the results into the desired threshold parameters.

3. *The outcomes have not been met and appear to be unlikely to be met given the current state of circumstances.* Remonitoring data are not significantly closer to the threshold parameters than in the initial study and may even be farther away.

In this case, the first step is to reevaluate what you are asking people to do. Whether they are staff, patients, vendors, other professionals, people generally wish to cooperate. When they are consistently resistant or noncompliant, it may be that what you are asking them to do is unrealistic. Determine if the standard to which you are holding them accountable is reasonable and appropriate. If the standard itself is the source of the problem, revise it. If, however, the standard is adequate, then evaluation of the appropriateness of the plan for the identified problem or opportunity should be undertaken.

Step 7 of the monitoring and evaluation process (Chapter 10) is revisited to determine if the etiology of the problem was correctly identified. A new analysis of the variance must be done to determine if a contributing variable might be responsible which may not have been identified during the indicator development process or if one of the identified contributing variables may be playing a more significant role than was previously thought. If so, an alternative plan may need to be developed. If not, all contributing variables must be identified and a new plan developed that addresses all of the contributing factors. For example, if a staff development plan to improve the nurses' compliance to documentation using nursing diagnosis fails to achieve its purpose, a staffing problem rather than ineffectiveness of the plan may be the cause. Questions to ask include the following:

- Is the standard a good one?
- Was the cause of the problem properly identified?
- Was the plan appropriate for the problem or opportunity?

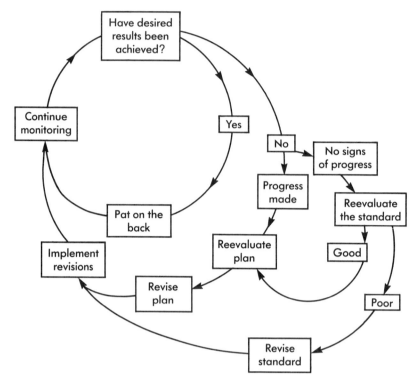

■ **FIGURE 12-2**   **Critical path of effectiveness analysis.**

- Did the plan address all of the contributing variables?
- If not, what other factors need to be addressed to resolve the problem or to take advantage of the opportunity?
- Should the plan be abandoned or merely revised?

If the plan must be abandoned, a new plan must be devised utilizing the strategies outlined in Chapter 11. If the plan simply needs revision, then a process review as outlined in step 2 above should be carried out and the necessary revisions made. The diagram in Figure 12-2 shows the relationship among the three options.

■ WHAT TO DOCUMENT

Documentation is frequently the benchmark by which quality is measured. It is an accreditation requirement and a legal necessity. Once written, the plan becomes evidence of the intent to act on an identified problem or opportunity. The process of implementation must also be documented. Process documentation involves recording what was done, when. Outcome documentation involves documenting progress.

Documentation may be broken down into three parts: data collection and analysis, planning, and evaluation. Data collection involves recording the collection of information. That information may be data regarding initial assessment or ongoing monitoring. Data may be clinical, professional, or administrative in nature. For example, recording the patient's vital signs over time is data collection, as is recording the number of nurses attending a continuing education event or the number of admis-

CRITICAL ISSUE	DATE	PROGRESS ENTRY	SIGNATURE

■ FIGURE 12-3   Progress record example.

sions, transfers, discharges, and deaths in a particular department for a particular shift. Data collection documentation also involves recording the implementation of routine activities such as turning patients every 4 hours or carrying out the essential activities listed in an action plan. Tools used to collect data usually take the form of flowsheets, which provide a quick summary of such things as numbers, activities, or symptoms over time. The data collection form (see Figure 9-1) is an example of a data collection flowsheet. Data collection is process documentation. The collected data must support the need for a plan of action. The analysis of the data provides that support.

Another form of process documentation is a plan. As mentioned earlier, it is the written record of the intent to act on a problem or opportunity. The tools used to record planning are the plans themselves. Plans are the second integral component of a comprehensive documentation system. Examples of plans are given in Chapter 11. The plan must delineate the results expected to be obtained once the plan has been implemented.

The third component of a good documentation system is evaluation. Documentation of evaluation is accomplished by keeping progress records, which serve as a diary of movement toward predetermined outcomes. Those outcomes are defined in the action plan. The tool most commonly used to document evaluation is the progress record. If the issue is clinical and involves patient care, progress toward patient outcomes is recorded. If the issue is professional, a staff progress record is required. A system progress record is required to follow the progress toward system outcomes as defined in the administrative action plan. Figure 12-3 is an example of a generic progress record. The critical issue may be a nursing diagnosis or patient problem if the plan is clinical in nature. It may also be an area for development if the plan relates to the staff, or a systems issue if the plan is administrative.

Data collection is used to diagnose the problem or opportunity. A plan of action is designed and implemented. Data regarding the effects of the action plan are gathered through remonitoring of the initial indicator so that an evaluation of change or progress toward the outcomes designated in the plan can be made. At each of these points, documentation is required. This documentation provides a record of:

- Quality problem or opportunity identification
- Planned strategy to address the problem or opportunity
- Implementation of that strategy
- Effectiveness of implementation

Whether the underlying problem or quality opportunity is clinical, professional, or administrative in nature, both process and outcome documentation are essential. Process documentation defines the problem and what is to be done about it; outcome documentation records the results achieved when the plan is implemented.

In conclusion, followup of the action plan requires evaluative judgment, i.e., the ability to evaluate the efficiency and effectiveness of the plan. The efficiency of the plan can be evaluated by using techniques such as cost-benefit analysis, while the effectiveness is analyzed by remonitoring the original indicator to identify quality improvement.

Documentation of data collection, action planning, and followup provides written proof of the quality improvement efforts and their results.

REFERENCES

1. Bleich M: Clinical judgments: essential elements of the nursing process, J Nurs Qual Assurance 4(4):1-6, 1990.
2. Bloom B et al: Taxonomy of educational objectives, handbook 1, cognitive domain, New York, 1956, David McKay.
3. An introduction to the Joint Commission nursing care standards, Chicago, 1991, Joint Commission on Accreditation of Health Care Organizations.
4. Lancaster J and Lancaster W: Concepts for advanced nursing practice: The nurse as a change agent, St. Louis, 1982, The CV Mosby Co.

13

STEP 10:
COMMUNICATING
RELEVANT INFORMATION

Everyone talks about communicating
but no one does anything about it.
MARK TWAIN

And they said: "Come let us build us a city, and a tower, with its top in heaven, and let us make us a name; lest we be scattered abroad upon the face of the whole earth. And the Lord came down to see the city and the tower, which the children of men builded. And the Lord said: "Behold, they are one people, and they have all one language; and this is what they begin to do; and now nothing will be withholden from them, which they purpose to do. Come let us go down, and there confound their language, that they may not understand one another's speech. So the Lord scattered them abroad from thence upon the face of all the earth; and they left off to build the city. Therefore was the name of it called Babel; because the Lord did there confound the language of all the earth; and from thence did the Lord scatter them abroad upon the face of all the earth.

Genesis 11:1-9

Nothing is more powerful than communication. Poorly planned and/or executed communication is like a tower of Babel—a hodge podge in which the right hand does not know what the left hand is doing.

Communication is the transfer of information from one person to another. Hamilton defines communication as the process of sharing thoughts, ideas, and feelings with others in commonly understandable ways.[3] Business communication refers to all of the oral and written information that is directly or indirectly applicable to the organization. Rosenblatt defines business communication as "purposive interchanges of ideas, opinions, instructions, and the like, presented personally or impersonally by symbol or signal as to attain the goals of the organization."[7] Step 10 of the Joint Commission's monitoring and evaluation process focuses on business communication. It is part of the internal operational communication, i.e., the structured communication that relates to achieving organizational work goals. Structured means it is built into the plan of operations—part of the routine communication that oils the organizational wheels. Typically, this type of communication is carried out through specific activities. For example, data collection reports, annual program evaluation reports, and quarterly trending reports may all be required communication.

■ CHARACTERISTICS OF BUSINESS COMMUNICATION

Communication is the lifeline of any business. Its significance cannot be over-estimated. Communication can be upward, downward, or lateral. It facilitates decision making at all levels, promotes understanding, and fosters organization and coordination. It is the culmination of hours of activity. Often the effects of work time are lost because its impact was poorly communicated. Frequently the reporting phase is viewed as anticlimactic and treated as an afterthought. Data are hurriedly slapped together and a brief summary of activity is generated. Communication, the most powerful tool available to influence decision making, is being used inappropriately and/or is underutilized.

Regardless of whether the communication is informal or formal, verbal or non-verbal, there are some common factors that bear on its success.

1. All communication must be receiver centered. In every communication, there is a sender and a receiver. The sender must understand the needs of the receiver and target the essence of the message to meet those needs. The receiver must understand the utility of the message if it is to be effective. For example, the possibility of contracting AIDS from an accidental needle stick makes the information regarding needle precautions extremely relevant to the practicing staff nurse.
2. Communication should be brief. The operant adage here is "Cut to the chase." What one has to say is only effective if it is heard/read and understood. Time is of the essence, so the quicker the point can be made, the more likely the receiver is to listen/read about the issue. Convey the main idea in as few words as possible.
3. Simple is better than complex. This goes hand-in-hand with brevity. KISS means "keep it simple and short." Choose the simple and straightforward over the complex and abstract.

■ PLANNING TO COMMUNICATE

Although much communication happens spontaneously, truly effective communication requires planning. Everyone at some point has been misunderstood or misinterpreted with unfavorable results. The key to success in outcome-driven communication is to focus on the desired results and plan the communication to achieve those ends.

Just as the lead paragraph in a newspaper article explains the five Ws (Who, What, Where, When, and Why), effective communication requires four Ws and one H. Before communicating, the sender must define:

1. *Who* needs to know about this?
2. *Why* do they need to know about it?
3. *How* is the message communicated most effectively?
4. *What* is appropriate to communicate?
5. *When* should the communication occur?

Each of these components translates into a distinct planning step.

Step 1: Who Needs to Know about This?

In this step you define your audience(s). There may be more than one individual or group who needs to receive your message. The question to ask is Who needs to know about the results of this QA study? Is it the staff? The nursing quality management council? The hospital-wide quality committee? Other departments? The audience is determined by three factors: First, those individuals or groups who are affected by the results should know about them. Second, administrative policy may outline who routinely receives communication regarding quality issues. Third, specific information may be generated that a particular group, which does not routinely receive this information, needs to act on. In this case, a special audience may be defined such as the executive committee or the board of directors, a hospital department, and/or a patient group.

Once the audience is determined, you can tailor the communication to your audience. Each individual or group approaches communication according to the individual's or group's current frame of reference. You should consider questions such as "Does this group have 'the big picture' or is it more concerned with a small piece of the pie?" According to Hamilton, since no two people have the same frame of reference, difficulty in communication is likely.[3] To avoid communication breakdown, it is necessary for the sender to understand the receiver's frame of reference. For instance, administrators frequently think in terms of cost and productivity and tend to have a broader frame of reference than staff. Staff often perceive matters personally, i.e., how will this information affect daily practice or individual responsibilities? Other departments view nursing messages from the perspective of their own discipline.

No two groups are alike, and it is the sender's challenge to identify the differences. What makes a particular group or individual unique? Do not overlook demographic variables such as age, sex, and academic preparation, or personality variables or styles such as commitment, authoritarianism, flexibility, and openness. The individual's or group's role or position in the organization may have a profound bearing on how communication is perceived. The vice president of nursing brings a different perspective than a new orientee. A group of patients may perceive information differently than would a vendor group. Tailoring communication to its intended audience is discussed more fully in step 4.

Audience analysis also includes a determination of how much the audience already knows about the subject presented and whether the receiver may have any preconceived opinions about the presenter. The credibility of the presenter can do much to facilitate or impede communication. An audience will listen to or read the words of a credible presenter and ignore a message presented by someone they do not respect. Hunt suggests using a worksheet to list important audience variables.[4] Figure 13-1 presents an example of an audience analysis worksheet.

Step 2: Why Do They Need to Know about It?

Typically, we communicate to inform, persuade, or recognize. Informational communication conveys data. It is the transmittal of facts and figures only. People in organizations need information to do their jobs. Dissemination empowers individuals and groups and enables them to make decisions and act on them. Rosenblatt suggests that business today "depends on a continuous supply of information, and a dependable distribution or communication system for both the receiving and delivering of the information messages to those responsible for making decisions and controlling operations."[7] An informational quality report is generated for specific individuals or

DEMOGRAPHIC CHARACTERISTICS

Age: Economic Status:

Educational Level: Political Status:

Occupational Type: Other Influences:

GENERAL AUDIENCE ATTITUDES

What are their political orientations?

What are their social orientations?

Where do they get their information?

What constituencies do they serve?

SPECIFIC AUDIENCE ATTITUDES TOWARD PROPOSAL

What do they think of your proposal?

Sources of their attitudes?

What attitudes can be changed?

What strategies may work?

SPECIFIC AUDIENCE ATTITUDES TOWARD COMMUNICATOR

What do they think of you?

What are your strengths (with listeners)?

What are your weaknesses (with listeners)?

Possible sources of credibility?

■ **FIGURE 13-1   Audience analysis worksheet.**
(From Hunt GT: Communication skills in the organization, ed 2, © 1989.
Reprinted by permission of Prentice-Hall, Englewood Cliffs, NJ.)

groups who need to keep abreast of the data generated by the monitoring and evaluation process; such groups might include the nursing quality management council or the hospital-wide QM council.

Directional communication is a type of informational communication. It provides instruction on how to perform specific activities or tasks. It enables people to learn how to accomplish desired outcomes.

While all reporting has an informational component, an informational report is generated for the data alone. Other types of communication use information to achieve specific ends. For example, the information in persuasive communication is used to influence, to motivate, or to control behavior in a predetermined way.

Persuasive communication is routinely used in health care. Convincing a staff member to work a double shift or a pediatric patient to take an unpleasant tasting medication requires persuasive skills. The objective of this type of communication is attitude change ultimately leading to behavior change.[6] Persuasive communication is a critical tool in reporting the results of monitoring and evaluation activities. It is the key to promoting the value of quality and may be the objective in reporting to the staff, administration, other departments, or any individual or group representing a barrier to quality improvement. Negotiation is a type of persuasive communication. The participants establish a common ground. Both sender and receiver may need to modify their attitudes/behaviors to achieve "a meeting of the minds." Ideally, the outcome is a win-win situation that is acceptable to all. Negotiation is a vital skill in communicating about quality management. However, many people are not comfortable negotiating or lack the necessary skills. There are many excellent references available to assist in developing or refining the requisite skills.

Recognition communication is essential to meet the social and psychological needs of workers. It motivates individuals to strive for continued growth. A pat on the back is only inches from a kick in the seat of the pants but miles apart in its effects. Unfortunately, quality assurance has traditionally been viewed as a mechanism for identifying problems and placing blame. However, recognition reporting is a particularly useful tool for acknowledging an individual's or group's achievement of or improvement in meeting quality goals.

A progress report may be generated to inform, persuade, or recognize achievements. It is a status update. A progress report provides a comparison of how things were and how they have changed. Are they better, worse, or the same? It may be concurrent, reporting how things are going, or retrospective, describing past performance. Fellows and Ikeda suggest that progress reports are worthless unless they address *why* something has changed. Without such an explanation, the report merely cites trends.[1] They advocate reporting the issue, the cause, the response, and the results. Quality reporting therefore must go beyond tracking and discerning trending. To be comprehensive, it must address the gamut of quality improvement efforts. Progress reports are part of the routine reporting within an organization.

As part of defining the purpose of the communication, you must also delineate the expected effect of your communication on the receiver. What are the desired outcomes of the communication? What impact will the communication have? Will knowledge improve? Will the receiver feel empowered? Will he, she, or they take action? What actions will be taken? Will attitudes and behaviors change? Which behaviors or attitudes will change? Will the receiver feel rewarded and appreciated? Defining the expected outcomes is critical because the content of the message will change based on the results to be achieved.

A cardinal error made by many professionals is providing different groups having different frames of reference with the same report. Typically, one report is generated and circulated to everyone on the routing list. Step 4 in the planning process targets the content to the receiver.

Step 3: How Is the Message Communicated Most Effectively?

This step deals with the channel through which the message is communicated. The two major channels are verbal and written, and both channels are either informal or formal. A "one on one" conversation about the results of a monitoring study between a head nurse and the department representative may describe informal verbal communication, while a verbal presentation to the board of directors about the status of quality improvement efforts requires a formal approach. A written communication to one department regarding a particular study may be handled through a memo, while the annual departmental quality report is a formal document.

There are advantages and disadvantages to both modes of communication. Verbal communication provides an opportunity for immediate feedback, while written does not. The written mode, however, enables the receiver to pace himself or herself for maximum comprehension, while the verbal mode does not. Written communication is more likely to be carefully thought out; verbal communication is typically more spontaneous.

Hamilton suggests six factors to consider in deciding which mode to use[3]:

1. The importance of the message
2. The needs and abilities of the receiver
3. How much and how soon feedback is needed
4. Whether a permanent record is required
5. The cost of the mode
6. Whether formality or informality is required

Sometimes the situation requires a combination of oral and written communication. For example, written handouts usually enhance a verbal presentation. Vardaman lists the key situations in which oral, written, or combined communication is most desirable[9] (Figure 13-2).

Once the medium has been determined, attention is turned to what is to be communicated and how it is to be presented.

Step 4: What Is Appropriate to Communicate?

When you have completed the above steps, you are ready to tackle the mountain of data, analyses, and quality improvement results you need to communicate. The challenge is to develop order within the information. First you must determine the appropriate content for each receiver. Not everyone who requires information needs the same information at the same depth. Steps 1 and 2 targeted the audience. Step 3 targets the format. Step 4 targets the message itself. What should be conveyed? Content that is appropriate for one audience may be inappropriate for another. Appropriateness is defined as suitability or fit for a particular use. Assessing appropriateness requires determining how the particular audience will use the information provided. The content should be tailored accordingly. If, for example, the purpose of the communication is to persuade the clinical practice council to reevaluate the falls-prevention program and action is the desired result, then the information presented in the

ORAL	WRITTEN	COMBINED
1. Confidential matters	1. Impersonalization desired	1. "Carry home" ideas
2. Warmth, personal	2. Extension in time and	desired
qualities needed	space proper	2. Follow-up needed
3. Open atmosphere	3. Storage and retrieval	3. Optimal undertanding
desired	needed	needed
4. Stronger feelings needed	4. Reliability/validity	4. Clarity and impact needed
5. Exactitude/precision not	important	5. Exploratory communication
required	5. Idea verification/authenti-	6. Audience participation
6. Immediacy required	cation needed	needed
7. Crucial situations	6. Objective references	7. Abstract/remote ideas
8. Added receiver impact	needed	
needed	7. Writing more acceptable	
9. Personal authentication	8. Crucial decisions/actions	
needed	9. Review/reconsideration	
10. Meeting social needs	needed	
	10. Supplement to speaking	

■ FIGURE 13-2   Summary of conditions for communication form.
(From Vardaman G: Effective communication of ideas, New York, 1970,
Van Nostrand Reinhold. Used with permission.)

communication must convince the council to act on your suggestion. If, on the other hand, the purpose of the message is recognition for meeting the quality targets set for pain management and the desired outcome is maintenance of performance, then the message must reinforce the desired behaviors.

Once the content for each audience has been identified, content must be arranged in the sequence it will assume in the report. A content outline is usually most helpful. Arrange the content outline from most important to least. If time is at a premium, the main points of the message will be delivered to the receiver in the first few minutes. Lesikar describes three types of sequencing: logical, direct, and chronological.[5] Logical sequencing uses inductive order, i.e., it moves from the known to the unknown. The facts are presented and then analyzed, and conclusions are drawn. In direct sequencing, deductive order is used. Conclusions are presented first, then the facts and analysis from which they are drawn. Chronological sequencing presents the findings in the order in which they occurred. It gives an historical perspective.

When constructing a content outline, remember the KISS principle: keep ideas as short and simple as possible without sacrificing the intent of the message. A general rule of thumb is that the length of the report is directly proportional to the severity of the problem it addresses. The more severe the problem, the more formal the report should be. According to Lesikar,[5] an outline should:

- Organize information to maximize understanding
- Show relationships among the pieces of information to be included
- Make the information fit together logically in the reader's mind

Keeping it simple also means selecting words that the audience understands. Avoid a long word when a short one will do. Use everyday language that the audience can relate to. Avoid using jargon or unfamiliar words.

When the audience is heterogeneous, with different levels of knowledge about the issue, or when the audience's academic preparation varies, the message must be aimed at the lowest knowledge level to avoid miscommunication.

Once the outline is generated, it provides the skeleton upon which to hang the meat of the report. In constructing the report, use active, rather than passive, verbs. Active verbs show the subject of the sentence doing the action. Passive verbs show the subject being acted upon. For example, "the staff of 4W reduced the incidence of level III medication errors by 10%" is a more powerful message than "the incidence level III medication errors have been reduced by 10% by the staff of 4W." Not only is the first version clearer, it is also shorter.

Choose precise words that convey an accurate description. A precise message leaves little room for misunderstanding and misinterpretation.

Keep sentences short. Long sentences are more difficult to understand than short ones. They tend to be less clear. Convey one idea per sentence. Lesikar suggests that sentences be bite sized.[5] A chunk of food that is too big is difficult to swallow. Similarly, a sentence that is too long is difficult to understand. Shorter sentences communicate more effectively.

■ PLANNING VISUAL AIDS

A picture is worth a thousand words. Graphic displays enhance all reports; however, they rarely can tell the whole story. Irvin S. Cobb stated "Don't tell me that one picture is worth a thousand words. Sometimes it's not worth one word. If I'm drowning, what do I do—hold up a picture? Hell no, I yell 'Help!'"[1] Do not allow visual aids to detract from the message. Choose them wisely.

Visual aids should clarify, i.e., they should help the audience understand the content. Many people do not like to read numbers and much information to be reported in quality reports involves numbers. Graphs and tables are useful tools for presenting quantitative data. They enable the reader to visually compare and contrast data.

There are four principles to keep in mind in using graphics.

1. Use them only when they are needed, i.e., when they clarify data or facilitate presenting a large quantity of data in a limited space.
2. Prepare the reader for the visual aid, i.e., tell the audience members that they are about to view a graphic aid.
3. Explain what it is.
4. KISS: Keep it short and simple.

Charts, graphs, and tables break up the content and can enhance visual interest. People are accustomed to visual depictions. They are pervasive in contemporary life, from the newspaper to the TV. We are bombarded with visual images.

The most common types of graphic aids include graphs and tables. A graph shows how pieces of data are related. It compares different classes of data. There are several types of graphs: the line graph, the bar graph, and the pie graph.

A line graph connects points on a scale to show trends. It depicts a change in some variable over time. Plotting the results of monitoring and evaluation activities on the threshold parameter tool and connecting the dots (Figure 13-3) is an example of a line graph. Typically the bottom line (horizontal axis) represents time and the side line (vertical axis) represents the variable that is expected to change over time.

Bar graphs depict relationships between two variables. Like a line graph, a bar graph may show change over time or it may compare two other variables such as the

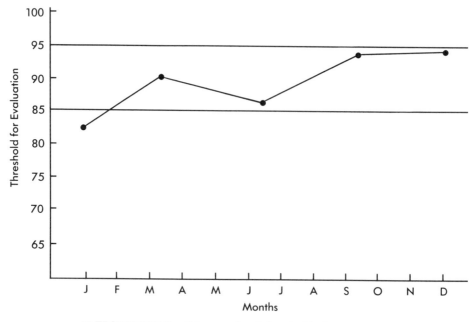

■ **FIGURE 13-3**   **Line graph of thresholds for evaluation.**

relationship of the QA results on a particular indicator by unit or by month. The differences within the data are shown by variations in the length of the bars. Figure 13-4 gives two examples of bar graphs. Bars may be horizontal or vertical but each bar must be labelled. As in the line graph, there is a vertical and a horizontal axis, each representing a distinct variable being compared.

A pie graph depicts proportions. It depicts the phenomenon being analyzed in the form of a pie. A wedge of the pie is assigned to each of the components that make up the pie. Each wedge represents a percentage of the total item being analyzed, and differences are shown by the sizes of the wedges. Slice the pie moving clockwise showing the pieces in descending order of magnitude. Figure 13-5 is a pie graph representing the percentages of clinical, administrative, and professional indicators to be monitored.

A table is an orderly arrangement of data. The data are arranged vertically in columns and horizontally in rows. Both columns and rows must be labelled. Tables are often used to clarify the relationships and meaning of the numbers. A table is an excellent mechanism for depicting large amounts of numerical data in a relatively small space. If particular numbers require special explanation, they should carry an asterisk or otherwise be marked, and a footnote should be added at the bottom of the table. The numbers for a generic screen might be represented in tabular form (Figure 13-6).

Lesikar outlines five general rules for effective table construction[5]:

1. If rows are very long, repeat the row heads on the right side.
2. Use a dash or an abbreviation such as "n.a." (not applicable) rather than a zero when data are not available.
3. Key footnote references to numbers in the table with asterisks or other unambiguous, nonnumeric symbols.

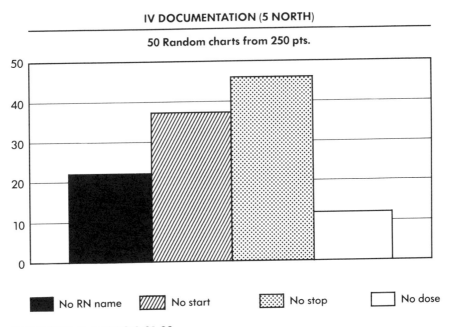

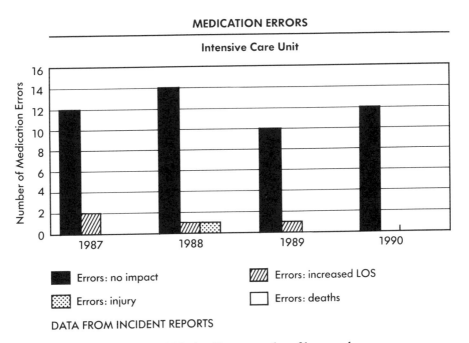

■ FIGURE 13-4   Two examples of bar graphs.

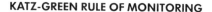

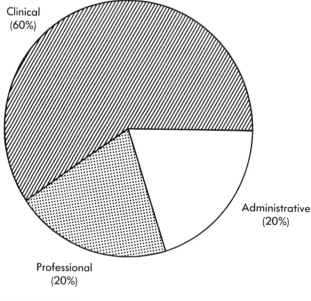

KATZ-GREEN RULE OF MONITORING

Clinical (60%)

Administrative (20%)

Professional (20%)

60-20-20 RULE

■ FIGURE 13-5   Example of a pie graph.

4. Include totals and subtotals whenever they enhance the value of the table. Columns and/or rows may be totalled.
5. Make clear the units in which the data were measured (e.g., years, months, dollars, clinical units).

Color is useful to highlight contrasting information. Using different colors for the lines, bars, wedges, or columns helps the reader compare the data.

Step 5: When Should the Communication Occur?

Timing is crucial. The practicability and desirability of acting on the communication depend on appropriate timing. The best planned communication is wasted if it is poorly timed. The likelihood of the receiver attending to what is presented and thinking about the information is determined not only by how but also by when the information is presented.

Vardaman lists four checkpoints to use in assessing communication feasibility: (1) situational conditions, (2) resource availability, (3) data adequacy, and (4) programming with other communications.[9] Situational conditions include timing, significance, credibility, and realism.

Bad news should never be delivered "cold" nor should an idea for radical change. It is important to time the communication for presentation when the receiver is most likely to be open to and to comprehend its significance. For example, administrators often are more receptive to the ideas of quality professionals immediately before and after a JCAHO site visit.

PATIENT FALLS
(Jan. 1, 1990, to December 31, 1990)

	Stage I	Stage II	Stage III	Stage IV
ICU/CCU	1	0	1	0
NICU	0	0	0	0
DETOX	5	2	4	2
OB/GYN	0	0	0	0
ONCOLOGY	2	1	3	2
MED-SURG	7	0	8	3
PEDS	11	2	14	3

Stage I: Witnessed, no injury
Stage II: Witnessed, injury
Stage III: Unwitnessed, no injury
Stage IV: Unwitnessed, injury

■ FIGURE 13-6   Example of a table.

Are sufficient fiscal, human, or material resources available to support the communication? If not, the content of the message would be moot. These resources must be secured before communication can occur.

Are the data sufficient to build the case? Has the change been in effect long enough to demonstrate the desired results? If not, the message may be premature.

Finally, the message must blend with other communications if it is to be successful. Receiving the report when other issues are consuming most of an individual's attention diminishes the force of the communication and decreases the likelihood of its being understood. Timing involves knowing who else in the organization is communicating what and to whom, and how your report is enhanced or diminished by these other communications. Sometimes "piggybacking" reports of a similar nature can strengthen the grouped reports, and the synergy among them can increase the likelihood of a positive response to each.

■ WRITING EFFECTIVE REPORTS

Written reports are probably the most common form of communication in organizations. Of course, they are effective only when they are read and understood. With the volume of paperwork that each administrator faces, the likelihood of a report being read is inversely proportional to the number of other reports in the administrator's "in" box. The busier a person is, the more likely he or she is to take reading shortcuts. Staff are now busier than ever. Long-drawn-out reports full of statistical analyses are likely to be scanned rather than read. One must never assume that because a report was written and distributed, it was read, even if reading it was requested or required.

Using the techniques suggested earlier in this chapter will yield a more effective report. Below are a few more suggestions to enhance the readability of a written presentation.

Reports have a greater impact when they are organized and presented appropriately. A written report represents the thoughts and work of the writer. It is a visual representation of its creator. When readers judge a report, they are considering not only the content but also the appearance of the work. In fact, the reader's impression of the content may be positively or negatively affected by the look of the report. A sloppy, disorganized report may suggest poorly developed, illogical ideas, while a well-organized and carefully formatted report may contribute to the credibility of the content.

Always include a cover sheet that identifies the title of the report, the date submitted, to whom the report is directed, and who prepared the report. Even if the report is merely a brief summary sheet, a cover sheet should be used. If the report is lengthy (e.g., >15 pages), include an abstract at the head. The abstract should be no longer than one page and should include the key points of the report. This way, a hurried reader can get the message quickly and return to the full report to digest the particulars as time permits.

Number all pages, figures, and appendices. There is nothing more frustrating to a reader than not being able to find a reference, figure, or chart. When possible, include the chart or figure in the body of the work so the reader does not have to flip back and forth between the pages.

Double check spelling and grammar. Excellent computer programs are available to check spelling and grammar. If these are not available, a dictionary should be consulted. If your report is important and especially if it is also lengthy, you should consider having someone else read it to identify grammatical or spelling errors before you finalize and distribute the report.

■ DELIVERING AN EFFECTIVE ORAL PRESENTATION

Most individuals fear public speaking. The mere suggestion of an oral presentation is enough to induce palpitations, sweaty palms, and a dry mouth. While much communication is written, sometimes an oral report is needed. The presentation may take the form of an informal briefing at a staff meeting or more formally as a report given at a council meeting or to an administrative group.

Many of the techniques described earlier in the chapter are useful in preparing a successful oral presentation. In addition, a few key points are given below.

In a written report, the writer is behind the scenes. In an oral one, the speaker is part of the message. The audience takes in both the message and the speaker's delivery and appearance. How they perceive the speaker can have a tremendous effect on how they relate to the message being conveyed. An anxious, disorganized, or unenthusiastic presenter can negatively affect the audience's perception of the speaker's competence and credibility, thus discrediting the message, too. A confident, enthusiastic, informed speaker can enhance the impact of the message.

There are two ways to deliver a verbal message: speaking one-on-one to an individual or delivering the message to more than one individual. When a message is conveyed one-on-one, it is a conversation. When it is delivered to a group, it may be thought of as an expanded conversation. An expanded conversation is merely an economical way of communicating the same message to many individuals.[7] To diffuse the panic associated with speaking before a large group, look for ways to reduce the presentation to a conversation. Seek out a friendly face. Initially, talk to that person. After about a minute, make eye contact with someone else and speak to that person for a little while. Move from face to face. Should you encounter an uninterested face, return to a friendly one for a confidence boost.

By and large the biggest mistake most novice presenters make is to read their work. An effective oral presentation is not a recitation. Think back to when you enjoyed being read to. Probably it was when you were a child, just before bedtime. No wonder audiences dislike being read to—it makes them feel childish and sleepy. Even the finest content may be destroyed by being read. If you need help remembering key points, write key phrases on note cards and number them to indicate the proper sequence. Show the major points on an overhead, slide, or flip chart so you do not lose your train of thought, but *never* read.

Preparation is the key to effective content and practice is the key to effective delivery. Rehearse, rehearse, rehearse. It will free you from clutching a prepared script as a life preserver.

Another important point to remember is that the brain can absorb only what the seat can endure. Many people become fidgety during presentations. Individuals listen more closely if the message relates to them. Relate the utility of the content for the audience early in the presentation, within the first 5 minutes if possible. This helps to set the stage for the information that follows. Another hint to set the stage for your presentation and to increase the likelihood of being heard is to eliminate environmental distractors. It is difficult to be heard in the midst of telephones ringing and beepers beeping. If the presentation is a planned formal one, choosing a site that minimizes disturbances of this kind is crucial. You do not want the VP to be beeped just as you are reaching the climax of the presentation.

Last, do not take yourself or your content too seriously—and do not forget to smile.

■ ADDITIONAL COMMUNICATION MECHANISMS

Two other mechanisms can be used to enhance communication about quality activities: the quality bulletin board and the institutional newsletter.

Swindle maintains that nearly everyone reads bulletin boards and almost no one reads newsletters.[8] That is because the information placed on bulletin boards is seen as important to the individual's relationship to the organization. The bulletin board must be strategically placed and properly controlled. Newsletters, however, are often seen as folksy tidbits about individuals within the organization, births, marriages, retirements, and sports scores. Changing that view requires a commitment to include pertinent and relevant information regarding quality activities and the impact of those activities on the individual's daily practice.

Both bulletin boards and newsletters are excellent tools to inform and recognize individuals for their quality improvement efforts. We suggest dividing the bulletin board into six sections to help staff find information quickly.[2] These include sections on information about the department of nursing, other departments, and quality. The other three sections include a spot for staff meeting minutes, required reading, and the general unit personal and professional recognition communications such as thank you notes, promotions, and certifications. To control paper flow, each item should be dated with its posting date and its removal date. One person, typically the department secretary, is designated to post and remove items in a timely manner and to record in the quality notebook the names of those staff members who have not completed required reading.

Organizing an effective newsletter can also promote an important communication link between staff and the organization. A regular column related to quality can be used to educate staff about quality, to foster a culture of quality, to inform staff about significant monitoring and evaluation findings, and to recognize the staff's quality efforts. One way to ensure that staff get the message is to make the newsletter required reading on the bulletin board.

While step 10 is the final one in the monitoring and evaluation process, it also is the first step in identifying quality problems or opportunities. Communication of relevant results is only as good as the feedback that the report elicits. What impact did the communication have and what results did it evoke? Mechanisms must be put in place to enable individuals, nursing departments, other departments, councils, and administration to respond to the quality communication.

Everyone within the nursing division needs to be touched by the quality communication network. It is the lifeline of organizational growth and development.

REFERENCES

1. Fellows H and Ikeda F: Business speaking and writing, Englewood Cliffs, NJ, 1982, Prentice-Hall.
2. Green E and Katz J: Make your bulletin board a QA tool, RN 53(1):38-39, 1990.
3. Hamilton C, Parker C, and Smith DD: Communicating for results, Belmont, CA, 1982, Wadsworth Publishing.
4. Hunt GT: Communication skills in the organization, Englewood Cliffs, NJ, 1980, Prentice-Hall.
5. Lesikar RV: Business communication: theory and application, ed 3, Homewood, IL, 1976, Richard D Irwin.
6. Rappsilber C: Persuasion as a mechanism for change. In Lancaster J and Lancaster W, editors: The nurse as change agent, St Louis, 1982, CV Mosby Co.
7. Rosenblatt SB, Cheatam TR, and Watt JT: Communication in business, Englewood Cliffs, NJ, 1977, Prentice-Hall.
8. Swindle R: The business communicator, Englewood Cliffs, NJ, 1980, Prentice-Hall.
9. Vardaman G: Effective communication of ideas, New York, 1970, Van Nostrand Reinhold.

Part Three

MANAGING QUALITY IN YOUR QUALITY MANAGEMENT PROGRAM

14

DESIGNING A VALUE SYSTEM FOR QUALITY

There's a big difference between motion and direction.
ANONYMOUS

Jim Martin, the building superintendent, was so angry that his hands shook. He paced back and forth the length of his office. He had tried to calm himself and finish some paper work while waiting for Carl, the new maintenance man, but he was too agitated to sit still.

Jim had summoned Carl immediately after receiving the report. After only 10 days on the job, Carl had been removing all the skylights in the old factory wing of the complex. The report also stated that a large order had been placed for sheetrock and plaster. What nerve! It sounded as if he intended to remove the skylights and plaster the holes.

The company had replaced all of the skylights 7 years ago with ones made of a new noncorrosive alloy, at considerable expense, too, when they had remodeled and converted the old factory wing into specialty shops. But the expense was not the worst of it. What was most upsetting to Jim was that the skylights were mandated by the building code. What would the company do when the inspector came?

Suddenly, there was a knock on the door. Jim took a deep breath and said, "Come in." He braced himself for a painful interview. Affably, with a huge grin, Carl entered.

"You sent for me, boss?" he said as he crossed the room, hand outstretched.

Jim took his hand with reluctance. As they unclasped hands, he thundered, "What is the meaning of removing all the skylights in the old factory wing?"

"Well," Carl replied, "since they were installed when the building was built in 1928 to vent the old coal heating system and since they leak and ruin merchandise every time it rains, I thought we should get rid of them."

Struck with the common sense of it, Jim stared openmouthed, absorbing Carl's words. His instinct agreed before his mind capitulated. Before he could organize his thoughts to speak, Carl stated the clincher. "I'm sorry if I've done something wrong, boss, but it seems to me those skylights no longer serve a purpose and should be gotten rid of. . . ."

In today's health care organizations there are many obsolete "skylights," things that, in Carl's words, "should be gotten rid of." A good quality management program will help an organization get rid of obsolete "skylights" in health care. The goal of a quality management program is to evaluate and improve the organization's efficiency and effectiveness constantly. Unfortunately, continuous improvement is not always the outcome of a quality management program. Sometimes the program is used to maintain the status quo. Furthermore, to many, the quality management program has come to symbolize extra work, audits, and excessive paperwork. This was especially true in the 1960s and 1970s when quality assurance became associated with audits of details, whether or not there were significant concerns at stake. During the 1980s, the traditional approaches to QA began to change. Spiraling health care costs, an older and sicker population, an explosion of technology, and a nursing shortage were some of the driving forces behind the changes. Today, quality assurance is being replaced by quality management, which requires a system for managing the quality of health care delivered to patients, managing the quality of professional practice offered by staff members, and managing the quality of the system of governance of the organization.

The quality management program is organized based on the principles and components of quality management outlined in Chapter 3. Like any other department, the quality department needs a value system, an appraisal system, and a response system.

■ THE VALUE SYSTEM

The value system—quality standards—must be developed first. The authors recognize that writing standards for the quality management department is a new idea. Nevertheless this step is necessary if total quality management of the organization is the goal. Since a successful quality management program requires considerable resources, thorough planning is necessary in advance. Thorough systems, carefully designed, have not been the traditional method of developing and conducting quality programs in most health care organizations. While health care organizations have traditionally developed standards to direct a program of patient care, they have typically overlooked the standards necessary to direct a program of quality management. Furthermore, most organizations felt justified in neglecting quality management standards because there is little in the way of research to guide them. One helpful resource is The Joint Commission's 1992 accreditation manual, which addresses quality standards in its quality assessment and improvement section.

Mission, philosophy, goals, policies, outcomes, procedures, practice guidelines, documentation, and the monitoring plan itself serve as the standards related to quality. The Joint Commission thinks that these should be in place. The 1992 standard QA.1 states that the leaders set expectations, develop plans, and implement procedures to assess and improve quality.[1] In order to monitor the quality management department, standards must be in place. These standards then act as the benchmarks against which the appropriateness, efficiency, and effectiveness of the program is measured. This chapter describes the development of the standards—the value system—for the quality management department.

■ THE APPRAISAL SYSTEM

The second component of a well-planned quality management program is the appraisal system. This component involves monitoring and evaluating the quality standards that have been developed to define the program. The appraisal system for the quality management program is discussed in Chapter 15.

■ THE RESPONSE SYSTEM

The response system is the third component of the quality management model. It is the quality improvement phase. This is the phase in which improvements are made in the process and outcomes of the quality program. The response system is discussed in Chapter 16.

■ USING THE THREE SYSTEMS OF QUALITY MANAGEMENT

The three systems of quality management—value, appraisal, and response—extend to every aspect of the organization's life. Quality management is not a program created to monitor only those activities carried out at the bedside. Rather, it should be a department within the division of nursing that monitors and evaluates not only care, but also professional practice and governance. Quality is a means, not an end. It is not what the organization *hopes* to achieve, it is what the organization actually accomplishes.

THE BLUEPRINT can be used to organize the quality management department, just as it can be used to organize all departments within the division of nursing. The authors believe that the sum of quality in each domain—clinical, professional, and administrative—equals total quality. Therefore, the organization of the department of quality management must incorporate the three domains in order to achieve total quality. The outcome of this organization-wide effort should result in lowered costs of care, decreased lengths of patient stays, and increased professional satisfaction as nursing makes a positive impact on patient outcomes. When things happen the way they are planned to happen, outcomes are positive and costs are controlled. Costs are controlled because the resources associated with redoing unsatisfactory work are eliminated.

The exciting thing about a total quality management program is "that we, as nurses, can make a difference, can influence and direct change which improves patient care and job satisfaction."[2] As Kathy Finch stated in a May 1990 address to the Fourth National Conference of the Canadian Foundation for the Advancement of Psychiatric Nursing, "When less attention is placed on the structural, systematic approach and more on examining what we do for the purpose of getting better results, all kinds of barriers melt away and QA becomes an open road for opportunity and achievement."[3] Obsolete "skylights" in health care can be eliminated or changed when we focus on quality improvement. A well-organized, planned quality management program ensures that quality improvement is a continuous process, rather than a periodic inspection or audit.

■ ORGANIZATION OF THE QUALITY MANAGEMENT DEPARTMENT

A successful quality management program encompasses far more than mere "paper exercises" designed in the hope of fulfilling Joint Commission requirements. To achieve its goals, a quality management program requires careful planning and organization. THE BLUEPRINT provides a basis for the organization of the quality management department. The quality management department is like any clinical department or staff development department. The only difference lies in "staffing." The quality management department is "staffed" by the quality management council. This council organizes and runs the quality management department.

Before this council can properly manage quality, however, the department must be organized to incorporate the three systems for quality management.

Once the value system is developed and organized, the appraisal and response systems can be developed. The work of the quality management program cannot begin until the value system is in place. Attempting to write a "quality management plan" without first organizing the department of quality management's value system can result in lack of direction, frustration, and wasted resources.

■ THE VALUE SYSTEM OF QUALITY MANAGEMENT

A suggested organization of the value system of an organization is presented in Figure 14-1. The authors recommend that quality management program standards be organized into structure, outcome, process, and evaluation standards just as THE BLUEPRINT organizes the division of nursing standards. The value system of quality management begins with its structure standards. Structure standards include the mission statement for quality, the philosophy of quality, the goals, and policies. Outcome standards follow. Outcome standards are the expected results of the quality process standards. Process standards of the quality management department include procedures, practice guidelines, action-planning (which includes the Joint Commission's ten-step process) and documentation. Evaluation standards include the cost of quality, productivity, satisfaction surveys, and process review. Once the value system is outlined, each standard can be formatted using the framework of THE BLUEPRINT. The health care organization can then create a quality management manual.

VALUE SYSTEM OF THE DEPARTMENT OF QUALITY MANAGEMENT	
STRUCTURE	1. Mission of quality management 2. Philosophy of quality management 3. Goals and objectives of quality management 4. Policies of quality management
OUTCOME	5. Outcomes of the quality management program
PROCESS	6. Procedures used in quality management 7. Practice guidelines used in quality management 8. Action planning of quality management 9. Documentation of quality management
EVALUATION	10. Appraisal of the quality management program 11. Satisfaction surveys of the quality management program 12. Research on improved methods of quality management

■ FIGURE 14-1   Value system of the department of quality management.

■ THE QUALITY MANAGEMENT MANUAL

The use of an "operations manual" is important to the quality management program. It provides the organization with a thought-out, written, formally approved, and legitimate way of conducting the organization's quality management activities. The manual assembles important materials describing the program into one reference. Without such a manual, information may be scattered among many memoranda, oral agreements, reports, and minutes. The manual survives despite lapses in memory and employee turnover.[4] The organization of the value system presented in Figure 14-1 lists a suggested sequence for the major sections of the quality management manual.

The following discussions describe how to write the individual standards within the quality management department and how to incorporate them into a useful manual.

Writing and Organizing the Mission of Quality Management

The mission of quality management within an organization is of paramount importance. It is not a repetition of the division of nursing's mission such as "to provide quality care," nor is it a repetition of the division of nursing's philosophy such as "to foster an environment for continuous quality improvement." It is, rather, an explanation of the reason for the existence of the quality management department. Figure 14-2 shows a sample mission statement for a quality management department. The mission statement justifies the existence of the quality management program. It should be harmonious with and should support the organization-wide mission. Just as the mission statement of an organization explains why it exists, so the mission of the quality management program explains its purpose. Remember, the mission statement *is* a structure standard. It should be placed first in the quality management manual.

THE MISSION OF THE QUALITY MANAGEMENT DEPARTMENT IS TO PROVIDE:

- The division of nursing with a systematic, planned, organized method of data collection

- A system that continuously monitors and evaluates patient care, professional practice, and governance

- The organization with specific, timely, quantitative indicators to facilitate the evaluation of excellence

- Organized mechanisms for implementing immediate or continuous quality improvements

---

■ FIGURE 14-2   Mission statement of the quality management program.

CLINICAL

In the domain of clinical practice, we believe that:

• Every patient has the right to expect quality nursing care.
• Every patient has the right to expect ongoing, systematic monitoring of the care provided to him/her.
• Improvements in clinical standards result from ongoing review of the efficiency and effectiveness of those standards in daily practice.

PROFESSIONAL

In the domain of professional practice, we believe that:

• All employees want to do good work.
• Monitoring the efficiency and effectiveness of nursing services is the responsibility of each employee.
• Quality must be part of the daily work experience.
• Education about quality is a vital component of each worker's professional development.
• Quality assessment is facilitated by peer review.

ADMINISTRATIVE

In the domain of administrative practice, we believe that:

• Commitment to quality begins at the top and permeates the division of nursing.
• Adequate resources must be allotted to the pursuit of excellence within the division of nursing.
• Decisions affecting nursing services are made with a focus on the impact of the decisions on the quality of the service.
• Quality improvement cannot exist in an environment of fear.
• Open communication and feedback regarding the results of quality assessment is critical to the pursuit of excellence.

■ FIGURE 14-3   Philosophy of quality management.

Writing and Organizing the Philosophy of Quality Management

The philosophy of the quality management program consists of a statement of beliefs, concepts, and principles describing the ideas, convictions, and attitudes of the organization about quality.[6] It serves as a guide for action and an explanation of action.[5] The beliefs provide a basis for carrying out the mission of the quality management program. Keep in mind that the philosophy of quality management should be realistic, understandable, believable, and achievable.

The philosophy of quality management should be written and placed in the next section of the quality management manual. It should be reviewed at least every 3 years. Figure 14-3 shows a sample philosophy of a quality management department. Note that the philosophy of quality management is divided into clinical quality beliefs, professional practice quality beliefs, and administrative quality beliefs. Once the department's philosophy is established, the goals and objectives can be formulated.

Writing and Organizing the Goals of the Quality Management Program

The goals of the quality management program are derived directly from the philosophy. The goals describe how the philosophy will be achieved. Goals express the broad-based desires for the program. They comprise the next section of the quality

Goal 1: To develop a commitment to the pursuit of quality at all levels within the organization

Objectives:
• To host a quality leadership conference for all nurse managers in October of this year
• To schedule an executive retreat to reestablish a commitment to quality and design a strategic plan for priorities for improvement this year

Goal 2: To provide the resources necessary to monitor and improve the practice of nursing within the division

Objectives:
• To redesign the job descriptions within the nursing division to include specific responsibilities for quality
• To include the quality management department as a cost center within the division of nursing

Goal 3: To utilize quality as the basis for decision making regarding the delivery of nursing services

Objectives:
• To appoint the quality manager as a consultant member of the executive nurse council
• To develop a mechanism to solicit customer input regarding specific nursing care decisions

Goal 4: To foster an environment of trust, cooperation, and risk-taking

Objectives:
• To institute a system for anonymous incident reporting
• To implement a program to facilitate staff nurse generated patient care innovation

Goal 5: To provide nursing staff with timely and meaningful feedback regarding the quality of their care delivery

Objectives:
• To install a quality bulletin board in each nursing department
• To institute a quarterly staff meeting devoted entirely to quality
• To make quality an agenda item for each meeting of the executive nurse council and each department staff meeting

■ **FIGURE 14-4**   Quality goals and objectives of the administrative domain.

management manual. Each quarter, the division of nursing QMC should evaluate the goals of the quality management program to alter, update, or record progress toward meeting the goals.

Objectives, or outcomes, add specificity to the goals by delineating how the goals will be achieved. Like the philosophy, goals and objectives must be written for clinical, professional, and administrative issues. Figure 14-4 is a sample of goals written in the administrative domain with the accompanying objectives. Note that the five goals listed in Figure 14-4 were derived directly from the administrative philosophy of quality management shown in Figure 14-3. In actual practice, goals would be written in each domain to correspond to each philosophy statement.

Note that goals and objectives are dynamic. They are written expressions of the activities occurring within the division of nursing. More than one objective may apply to each goal. Formulating goals must not be a paper exercise undertaken solely to get through the accreditation process, but, rather, the creation of dynamic directives for quality improvement.

Writing and Organizing Policies for Quality Management

Policies, as defined in THE BLUEPRINT, are non-negotiable rules. Those rules governing the quality management program are maintained in the next section of the quality management manual.

Three types of quality management policies should be written: clinical quality policies, professional quality policies, and administrative quality policies. Remember, every organization is bound to its policies, so be wary of creating impressive quality management policies that would be impossible to implement with available resources.

Quality Policies in the Clinical Domain. Policies that govern quality management of patient care occupy this next section of the manual. These policies outline the non-negotiable rules of quality management in the clinical domain. In these clinical quality policies, each organization must state its own rules for governing the quality of patient care. The policies must be realistic and achievable, based on the organization's available resources. Publication of a complete outline of quality policies in this book is not feasible. However, examples include statements that quality management studies will be conducted by those involved in the care and that every study will use the trifocus approach of patient, staff, and system. Rules will be delineated in this section regarding the types of clinical quality studies to be conducted as well as the rules for conducting clinical trials and patient research within the organization. In short, any nonnegotiable rules of the organization directly pertaining to setting clinical standards, monitoring and evaluating patient care, and improvement in patient care will be maintained in this section.

Quality Policies in the Professional Domain. Quality policies in the professional domain include the nonnegotiable rules for monitoring the professional practice of the staff. These policies comprise the second division of the policy section of the manual.

Professional practice quality policies address key aspects of quality management in professional practice within the organization. These policies specify role responsibilities in quality awareness, appraisal, and improvement. For example, a policy may state that all members of the division of nursing must be involved in monitoring and evaluation activities.

Quality Policies in the Administrative Domain. The policies of quality management in the administrative domain are the nonnegotiable rules for managing quality in the system. The policies in this domain should specify responsibility and accountability for quality in the division of nursing. This section specifies the rules for data collection including how often data will be collected, the rules for tabulation of data, for data compilation, and reporting and archive requirements. For example, critical aspects of care must be monitored four times per year.

This section should also specify how often quality management standards will be reviewed and updated. In short, the "rules of the game" for quality must be outlined in an organized fashion and maintained in the quality management manual. Remember, however, that policies are nonnegotiable so develop them wisely.

Writing and Organizing Outcomes for Quality Management

Next the outcomes that the organization expects from its quality management program must be delineated. The written outcomes describe what the organization hopes to achieve by implementing a quality management program. Every organization wants to enhance the quality, appropriateness, and effectiveness of the delivery of patient care. In order to do that, the organization must first develop systems of evaluation of patient care, of staff performance, and organizational standards of quality. Every organization must develop its own standards or value system, its own quality assessment or appraisal system, and its own improvement mechanisms or response system. These systems provide the benchmarks against which quality will be measured and outcomes can be evaluated. Quality outcomes are incorporated into the process standards of the quality management department. For example, the outcome of the practice guideline for conducting a monitoring and evaluation study might be planned, organized, systematic ongoing studies based on department specific important aspects of care/service.

Writing and Organizing Process Standards for Quality

Process standards include procedures, practice guidelines, action plans, and documentation related to quality.

Procedures for Quality Management. All procedures of the quality management program should follow the same format. Included in the procedures of the quality

---

Title: Combine related issues in one procedure.

Personnel: List the types of staff allowed to perform this procedure.

Desired outcome: Describe the result you wish to obtain by having the staff follow the steps of this procedure.

Supportive data: Include only information needed or helpful to perform this procedure. It is not necessary to describe the procedure's rationale or purpose.

Tools, forms, and location: Describe items needed to perform the procedure and where to find them.

Steps:

1. Begin each step with an action verb.

2. Write steps in order of occurrence.

3. Illustrate and add diagrams for clarification.

4. If there is an associated practice guideline, include its initiation or discontinuation as a step.

Include any precautions related to the specific steps.

Include any alterations or modifications for special patients.

Include any patient explanations as required throughout procedure.

Do not include vague rationales.

Documentation: Describe what, where, and when documentation must be initiated.

Authors of procedure: List members of staff who wrote this procedure.

References: List resource person(s) or literature used in formulating the procedure.

Approval: Specify date and mechanism of original approval.

Review date: List anticipated review date (every three years).

Revision date: Copies must be archived when revised.

Distribution: Indicate whether this is generic or unit specific and which units must have it.

■ FIGURE 14-5   Procedure outline.

management department are explanations of how to carry out tasks or calculations such as standard deviation or data entry into a computer. Procedures are process standards. Like other procedures in the division of nursing, they describe psychomotor skills involved in quality management.

One suggested format that may be used to describe how to carry out the tasks of quality management is shown in Figure 14-5. These procedures are maintained in the

---

QUALITY MANAGEMENT DEPARTMENT

Title: Procedure for Patient Telephone Interview

Personnel: Nursing personnel or volunteer staff.

Desired outcome: To provide data about the degree of customer satisfaction with (a) nursing care, (b) professional practice, and (c) governance of the organization.

Supportive data: Telephone interviews provide retrospective data.

Tools, forms, and location: Use form A-2101, entitled "Discharged Patient Telephone Interview". This form is located in the blue manual, Section 4.

Steps:

1. Obtain patient discharge list.

   This list is available daily from medical records.

2. Call patients beginning at the top of the list.

   If no answer, note on list. Call may be repeated later at the discretion of the interviewer.

3. Request time and charge for each long distance call.

   Time and charge must be a verbal request to the operator.

4. Explain purpose of call to the patient.

   If met with resistance, pleasantly terminate the call.

5. Ask interview questions in order.

   Do not ad lib. Do not interject personal comments.

6. If a complaint is registered, promise a call back.

   Refer to appropriate person to answer complaint.

7. Place completed telephone interview forms in red manual.

   Red manual will be picked up and calls evaluated monthly at quality management council meetings.

Documentation: Document interview on form A-2101.
Document patient's name, phone number, time and charges in the telephone log.
Document positive, neutral, and/or negative responses on Quality Management Telephone Response Tally Sheet.

Authors of procedure: Quality Management Council

References: Katz, Jacqueline, RN, MS, Green, Eleanor, RN, BSN, Managing Quality, Mosby–Year Book, St. Louis, 1992.

Approval:

Review date:

Revision date:

Distribution: Volunteer Office, Same-Day Surgery, Clinic, Emergency Department, Dialysis Department.

■ FIGURE 14-6   An example of a quality management procedure.

quality management manual for easy access and reference. An example of a quality management procedure for patient telephone interview is shown in Figure 14-6. The authors recommend that quality management procedures be reviewed and updated every 3 years.

Practice Guidelines for Quality Management. Practice guidelines for the quality management department are written to direct staff members in the management of quality-related activities. Like clinical, professional, and administrative practice guidelines, quality management practice guidelines may be collaborative.

Practice guidelines provide an organization with a tool for standardizing quality management activities. They promote continuity in quality management practices from department to department and for new employees. Unlike policies, practice guidelines are negotiable. In other words, they provide direction while permitting modifications to be made when warranted by professional judgment.

When practice guidelines are implemented, things happen the way they are planned to happen in the quality management department. Practice guidelines are process standards. Figure 14-7 is an outline of a suggested format for a quality management practice guideline. Figure 14-8 illustrates a sample quality management prac-

---

Title: Specific Quality Management Situation

Personnel: List the types of staff permitted to implement these guidelines. Indicate if certain components may be performed only by certain levels of workers.

Critical competencies: Describe the knowledge or skills necessary to carry out this practice guideline.

Outcomes: Describe the specific result(s) you hope to achieve by implementing this practice guideline.

Indications: Describe the specific populations or situations for which this practice guideline is designed.

Areas of responsibility:	**Orders:**
1. Assessment	Use action verbs, e.g. change, check, assess, stop, notify, etc. List tools used and frequency of their use.
2. Planning	
3. Interventions	
4. Evaluation	
5. Documentation	Include information to be charted on each form and what pieces of information go on which form, how often the documentation should occur.

Authors: List author(s) of protocol.

References: List resource persons or literature used in developing this guideline.

Approval: Specify date and mechanism of original approval.

Review date: List anticipated review date.

Revision date: Copies must be archived when revised.

Distribution: Indicate whether the guideline is generic or unit-specific and which units must have it.

■ FIGURE 14-7   Quality management practice guidelines format.

MANAGEMENT OF VARIANCE

Personnel: Unit Quality Assurance Coordinators
Quality Management Council

Critical competencies: 1. Must have completed 3 hour in-service on the quality
management program.
2. Must have handled one prior variance under supervision
of a QA preceptor.

Outcomes: 1. Variations outside the confidence interval will be handled by
the quality management coordinator in a planned,
organized, systematic manner.
2. There will be continuity of handling variations within the
organization.

Indications: This practice guideline will be initiated when data fall outside the
organization's established confidence interval.

Areas of responsibility:	Orders:
1. Assessment	1.1 Assess the degree of variation— sentinel event or rate based indicator?
	1.2 Assess the seriousness of the variation.
	1.3 Assess the impact of the variation on the patient, staff, or system.
	1.4 Assess the cause of the variation.
2. Planning	2.1 Plan a course of action based on analysis: a. Second review b. Query review c. Intensive review
3. Interventions	3.1 Initiate further reviews.
	3.2 Take action to solve variation— initiate an action plan: a. Coordinated care plan b. Employee development plan c. Administrative action plan
4. Evaluation	4.1 Evaluate the progress of the action plans.
	4.2 Evaluate the impact of the corrective action on the patient, staff or system.
5. Documentation	5.1 Document analysis statement on confidence interval tool if variance detected from routine monitoring.
	5.2 If variation is a clinical outlier, document on the End-of-the-Shift Report.
	5.3 If variation is a sentinel event, document on an incident report.
	5.4 Document all reviews on QMC Tracking Tool.
	5.5 Document all interventions on the appropriate action plan.

Authors: Quality Management Council

References: Quality Management Council Quality Management Plan

Approval: _____

Review date: _____

Revision date: _____

Distribution: Unit Quality Management Manuals

■ FIGURE 14-8   Practice guideline for management of a variance.

tice guideline for management of a variance. Note that the format uses the nursing process. Other examples of practice guidelines might include how to conduct a monitoring study or how to develop an action plan for improvement.

Action Planning for Quality Management. Action planning for quality management has been given much attention by the Joint Commission. To provide guidance and to ensure some standardization from organization to organization, the Joint Commission developed a ten-step process. This ten-step process, when carried out by an organization, demonstrates quality management action planning. Action plans will be highly individualized for each organization because each organization will outline the tools and policies governing its own program.

Ideally, the written quality management plan should be maintained in the quality management manual in the section that follows the practice guidelines. Each organization must develop an individualized quality management plan that fits its unique situation.

Documentation of Quality Management. Documentation used within the quality department of the organization includes every tool, form, and chart used in quality management. Standardized documentation ensures consistency. For example, we recommend that one data collection tool be used throughout the organization. Furthermore, there should be one method employed to analyze and compile data. The method should be simple enough to enable colleagues from all departments to understand the data, interpret the results, draw conclusions, and act to create improvement.

The documentation used in the quality management program is the responsibility of the quality management council. It must be a carefully considered process rather than a haphazard assortment of forms and reports. Since data collection is the backbone of quality management, the importance of accurate documentation methodology cannot be overemphasized.

Some of the pieces of documentation which may be used in the quality management department are:

- Council structure chart
- Matrix for delineating scope of care and service
- Patient, staff, management profiles
- Matrix for recording important aspects of care/service
- Indicator development form
- Data collection tool/data analysis tool
- Threshold parameter tool
- End-of-shift report
- Justification of variation form
- Management rounds quality assessment form
- Suggestion forms
- Satisfaction survey forms
- Incident reports
- Quality management calendar

While this list may seem to represent a large volume of documentation, remember that quality management is a *department* and the documentation for the operation of a department cannot be accomplished with one or two forms. Quality management documentation must be a carefully considered process with one form building upon and complementing another.

Writing and Organizing Evaluation Standards for Quality

Evaluation standards in the quality management department consist of reviews of the processes involved in quality management at least quarterly, the satisfaction questionnaires and interviews of staff members relative to their satisfaction with the quality program, and clinical, professional, and administrative indicators of quality performance. For example, one clinical indicator of quality performance might be the number of patient care problems resolved by quality improvement efforts. An example of a professional indicator of quality performance might be the certification of every data collector. An example of an administrative indicator of quality performance might be the appropriation of funds to develop and maintain a quality management program within the organization.

Creation of a sound value system for the quality management department provides a solid foundation upon which to build the next two components of quality management—the appraisal and response systems. The authors remind readers that many of these concepts are new. While many organizations are struggling to define quality management programs relative to clinical care, few have identified the need to look within the quality management department itself first. The authors strongly believe that the quality standards must be in place first before any work can be done to improve the quality of patient care.

REFERENCES

1. Accreditation manual for hospitals, Chicago, 1992, Joint Commission on Accreditation of Healthcare Organizations.
2. Allen DG: The social policy statement: a reappraisal. Advances Nurs Sci 10(1):39-48, 1987.
3. Finch K: Quality assurance: the open road to excellence in psychiatric nursing. Speech presented at the Fourth National Conference-Canadian Foundation for the Advancement of Psychiatric Nursing, May 1990.
4. Juran M: Quality control handbook, ed 4, New York, 1988, McGraw-Hill Book Co.
5. Poteet GW and Hill AS: Identifying the components of a nursing service philosophy, J Nurs Admin 18(10):29-33, October 1988.
6. Yeaworth RC: The ANA code: a comparative perspective, Image J Nurs Schol 17(3):94-98, 1985.

15

EVALUATING YOUR
QUALITY MANAGEMENT PROGRAM

Here is a piece of advice that is worth a king's crown:
To hold your head up, hold your overhead down.

RUTH BOOSTIN

Long ago in a kingdom called Phrygia in the country of Turkey there lived a very foolish king. One day the king's servants brought to him a drunken satyr. Since satyrs spent all of their time with Bacchus, the god of wine, it was not unusual for a satyr to be drunk. After many days of partying with the satyr, the king decided to return him to Bacchus. In appreciation for the return of the errant satyr, Bacchus agreed to give the king anything he wanted. Being greedy, the king loved gold more than anything else, so he asked for the power to turn anything to gold simply by touching it. Bacchus knew this was a stupid request but he could not deter the king. "So be it. You have what you want."

The king was ecstatic for, in fact, everything he touched did indeed turn to gold. Flowers, rocks, his cloak, his shoes—everything he touched became gold. He would be the richest man in the world. By the time he returned to the palace he was tired and hungry; however, the bread turned to gold when he tried to take a bite. The wine turned to liquid gold when he tried to drink it. Unable to eat or drink and so heavily weighted with golden clothes and jewelry, the king returned to Bacchus and asked him to undo the gift.

The king was very embarrassed and looked so silly that Bacchus could not stop laughing. "Go to the River Pactolus and wash yourself. When you come out of the water, your power will be gone." So sick of gold was the king that he never wanted to see anything made of gold again.

The king in this story is Midas and variations on the story abound; however, there are really two major morals to Ovid's famous tale. One is that too much of a good thing can be too much and the second is that the cost of something may far outweigh its benefits. These morals have implications for the current popularity of quality programs in health care. This chapter focuses on analyzing those implications and discussing the appraisal of a quality management program. This chapter breaks new ground in that there has been little emphasis to date in the literature regarding some of the issues presented here.

In the past, quality management programs were perceived as luxuries which could be afforded when things were going well and the institution was operating "in the black." Today, they are viewed as a competitive advantage, an economic lifejacket for an institution floundering in a financial "Red Sea." Research indicates that businesses with higher quality and larger market share earn margins about five times greater than businesses with lower quality and smaller share.[13] *Hospitals* magazine recently reported that investors and credit agencies are beginning to examine the relationship between a hospital's financial performance and its quality of care.[10] The future role of quality management programs, however, is neither as a luxury nor as a lifesaver. It will not be an optional approach, nor will it be part of a crisis management strategy; rather quality management will be a routine function in health care. It will become a routine part of the operating system of every health care institution. Competing on the basis of quality will be part and parcel of everyday operations in health care. The most significant changes will take place in the focus of the quality management program, which will shift from problem identification and resolution to improvement. Garvin states, "In my view, most traditional principles of quality were narrow in scope; they were designed as purely defensive measures to pre-empt failures or eliminate defects. What managers need now is a strategy to gain and hold markets with quality as a competitive linchpin."[8] Dr. Deming states, "Inspection with the aim of finding the bad ones and throwing them out is too late, ineffective and costly. . . . Quality comes not from inspection but from improvement of the process."[18]

This new thrust in quality improvement requires a reevaluation of many existing programs with some redesign, too. Typically, program evaluation is conducted to facilitate decision making regarding the viability of a program. This will not be the case with quality programs, which will soon be essential in all health care institutions. Rather, the purpose of quality program evaluation is to determine the appropriateness, efficiency, and effectiveness of the quality efforts. In the future, directors of quality programs and department managers responsible for department-based quality management programs must provide the most cost-effective means for monitoring and improving quality. An evaluation of that process is necessary. David Burda in the cover story of the January 28, 1991, issue of *Modern Healthcare* states that total quality management has become an umbrella term for strategies that "identify and meet customer expectations, reduce the cost of non-compliance with standards, strive for 'zero' defects, reduce outcome variability, eliminate the cost of poor quality, use statistical methods to identify and monitor processes and continually work for improved quality."[3] He adds that while total quality management has become big business in health care, it may actually be adding substantially to operating costs, "the precise ailment that total quality management is supposed to cure."[3]

Carroll suggests that there are two basic reasons for an annual formal review of the quality management program. The first reason is to determine the cost effectiveness and productivity of the program and the second reason is to meet Joint Commission requirements.[4]

▪ QUALITY PROGRAM EVALUATION

Program evaluation involves the process of identifying specific kinds of information that interested parties would need in order to make decisions about the program. The process includes collection, analysis, interpretation, and dissemination of that information to the appropriate audience.[16] Project evaluation was discussed in Chapter 12. This includes the analysis that is undertaken for each important aspect of care that the department monitors. Many quality monitoring projects make up the total quality management program. However, quality program evaluation is more than the sum of all the project evaluations. It involves a formative and summative review of the quality management program itself.

Accrediting bodies may require a program evaluation, or the administrative body of the organization may require it to make decisions about the status of the program. The 1992 Joint Commission Standard QI.5.1 requires an annual comprehensive report on the evaluation of quality improvement activities.[1]

As with any quality study, indicators are used as barometers to judge program soundness. Four areas of indicator development are necessary to evaluate the quality management program: cost, productivity, processes, and satisfaction. Evaluating the quality management program requires both process and outcome review and efficiency and effectiveness analysis. Efficiency deals with the processes and effectiveness deals with the results or outcomes. Process review provides information about the efficiency of the quality management program while analysis of cost, productivity, and satisfaction measures its effectiveness.

To provide a comprehensive review of the quality management program, each of the four areas cited above must be analyzed. However, traditional approaches to quality assurance program evaluation have focused primarily on a process review. Although some attempts have been made to identify the impact of monitoring and evaluation activities on the quality of patient care, very little information is available on cost. In light of this, the authors suggest some preliminary measures that can be used to quantify the effectiveness of a quality management program. It is our intent to stimulate further thought about the development of indicators that define the quality of a quality management program.

■ QUALITY PROGRAMMING—THE GOLDEN TOUCH?

Some health care organizations value their quality programs as much as King Midas valued gold. In fact, the results that can be realized by initiating quality management may be just short of miraculous; however, the cost of achieving those results must be considered.

Quality and cost are inextricably linked. Donabedian describes the relationship between quality and cost as follows[6]:

1. Quality costs money.
2. Money does not necessarily buy quality improvement.
3. Some improvements in quality are not worth the added cost.

Quality is desirable. Quality is essential. But quality at any cost is foolish. Juran identified that quality could be understood in terms of avoidable and unavoidable costs. Avoidable costs result from defects and product or service failures. Unavoidable costs are associated with prevention, i.e., inspection, sampling, sorting, and other quality-control initiatives. To Juran, the failure costs were "gold in the mine" because they could be retrieved by quality improvement efforts.[12]

Crosby defines the cost of quality as the expense of nonconformance. He divides that cost into prevention, appraisal, and failure categories and suggests that 15% to 20% of income is often spent in these three areas.[5]

Prevention costs are those associated with activities designed to prevent problems in the development of a product or service. In the case of hospitals, this would apply to the standards development phase. Examples would include the cost of writing the standards; the cost of educating staff about establishing standards of excellence; the cost of learning to use the tools associated with monitoring; and the cost of improving those tools.

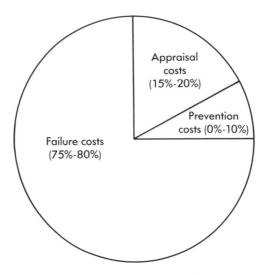

■ FIGURE 15-1   The costs of quality.

Appraisal costs are those incurred during the monitoring and evaluation phase. These would include the costs of staff hours for data collection and analysis, the quality management council's time in designing the divisional monitoring and evaluation plan and reporting inspection results. Appraisal costs can account for more than 15% of total quality costs.

Failure costs are easily identifiable. They are the costs of doing things incorrectly. They reflect the difference between what it costs to manufacture a produce (reality) and what it would cost if there were no failures during manufacturing (ideal situation). Actual manufacturing dollars minus ideal manufacturing dollars equals failure costs. Israeli and Fisher report that failure costs account for 75% to 80% of the total quality costs in most organizations. They state that reducing failure costs will also reduce the appraisal costs.[9] Figure 15-1 illustrates the relationship of the three components of quality cost.

Included in these costs are the labor and materials required for the initial work and rework as well as the opportunity costs associated with the rework. For example, the cost of restarting an IV because of poor technique is three times that of doing it correctly the first time. First, there is the cost associated with the initial attempt, i.e., the nurse's time and the equipment. In addition, there is the cost of the rework, i.e., the additional nurse's time and the equipment required to restart the IV. Finally, there are the opportunity costs, i.e., the nurse's time because he/she could have been doing something else during the time taken to redo the work not done correctly initially.

Most readers will agree that the cost of quality is a critical factor to consider in examining patient care. Quality improvement programs are geared to focus on the failure and prevention costs but few have looked closely at the appraisal costs. Assuring that "the golden touch" does not become a costly nightmare requires a realistic approach to evaluating the true worth of your quality program.

Quality costs must be identified and quantified to determine if they fall within an acceptable range. Frequently, quality department directors and nursing department managers have no idea how much they spend on quality. Crosby believes that a well-run quality management program can get by with spending less than 2.5% of operating income on quality and suggests that most of those dollars should be spent on prevention and appraisal.[5]

■ DETERMINING COSTS ASSOCIATED WITH QUALITY

Cost analysis involves examining the quality management program in relation to its cost. There are three elements of cost which should be considered: labor costs, materials costs, and overhead costs. Labor costs include the cost of the time of those staff members involved directly in quality management activities. These can include data collection activities, committee meetings, educational activities, report writing, action planning, and piloting change.

To calculate labor costs, the amount of time staff spends in quality activities must be assigned a monetary value. First, the percentage of time each individual staff member spends on quality management is estimated. Then that percentage is multiplied by the individual's salary and fringe benefits to determine the direct labor costs. For example, if 5% of a staff registered nurse's time is spent in quality activities and his or her annual salary is $35,000 + $7,000 in fringe benefits, the computation would be:

$$0.05 \times \$42,000 = \$2,100 \text{ spent in quality activities}$$

If that department employs 15 nurses, each of whom devotes 5% of his or her time on quality activities, the annual direct labor costs for quality activities would be $31,500 per year. Additional estimates for other types of staff would furnish similar dollar amounts. All the labor costs should be added to yield an annual total for each department. The totals from each department are then added, to yield the total labor costs associated with quality in the division of nursing.

Dividing the total labor costs per department by the number of important aspects of care being monitored in each department calculates the average labor cost incurred for the quality management program related to each aspect of care:

$$\frac{\text{Total labor costs}}{\text{Number aspects monitored}} = \text{Average labor cost per aspect monitored}$$

Dividing the total labor costs for the division of nursing by the total number of different indicators being monitored throughout the division of nursing would yield the cost per indicator. It is important to note that this figure may be higher than the individual department labor cost per aspect of care since more than one department may be monitoring the same important aspect.

Materials costs include the costs of supplies necessary to carry out the quality management activities. These costs are usually easy to quantify. They include the costs of supplies associated with standards development and monitoring and evaluation activities, as well as the cost of typesetting and duplicating forms, telephone charges, audiovisual materials and equipment used, computer software and supplies, binders, promotional or motivational materials, and the like.

Materials costs also include supplies and equipment associated with problem correction or quality opportunity development. For example, if improving patient outcomes and satisfaction for pain management requires the purchase of additional patient-controlled analgesia units, that cost should be considered when analyzing the cost of quality. Materials costs therefore may vary significantly upward or downward depending on the quality improvement activities that occur from year to year. These costs added to direct labor costs equal the direct program costs.

The direct costs divided by the number of important aspects being monitored yields information about the aspects-specific costs. Analysis of the components of direct costs may reveal ways to reduce them. For example, if a significant percentage of the nurse's time is spent in data collection, perhaps reassigning that activity to a lower-salaried worker could reduce the cost of gathering data.

Overhead costs include those associated with indirect labor. That is, employees who do not work on the end product but provide services related to production. For example, the cost of additional staffing necessary to relieve staff for quality management activities is an indirect cost. Overhead also includes fixed and miscellaneous costs such as office space, utilities, senior level management, divisional quality coordinator, and facilities maintenance. Usually a fixed amount for overhead is determined by averaging costs or by calculating a percentage of direct labor costs.

Determining overhead is an indirect estimation. Often it is allocated at the same rate as that of direct labor. Therefore if 2.5% of direct labor costs are allocated to quality initiatives, 2.5% of the department's overhead may be allocated as related to quality. Also, some organizations allocate a percentage of the divisional overhead to each department. If so, a percentage of this overhead may also be included when estimating overhead associated with quality. A quick consultation with the finance department will help to identify the actual figures associated with overhead and will also uncover any accounting idiosyncrasies that might modify the cost of quality equation. Therefore, the authors suggest utilizing the finance department as a resource in calculating cost of quality.

The sum of direct labor costs, materials costs, and overhead costs is the total cost associated with quality. As stated earlier, Crosby recommends that the total cost not exceed 2.5% of operating income.[4] As with thresholds, however, the authors believe that it is difficult to hit a pinpoint target. We, therefore, suggest setting an acceptable range for total quality costs. Also, because we are including the costs associated with quality improvement in the total quality costs, the authors suggest a range of about 2.5 to 4.5%. To calculate this percentage, divide the total quality costs by the total operating income and multiply the result by 100%.

$$\frac{\text{Direct costs (labor costs + materials costs) + Overhead costs}}{\text{Operating income \$}} \times 100\% = 2.5\text{-}4.5\%$$

If total labor costs for quality activities were $31,500, the materials costs were $10,000, and overhead costs were $2,000 for a department with an annual operating income of $1,100,000, the calculation would be as follows:

$$\frac{\$31,500 + \$10,000 + \$2,000}{\$1,100,000} \times 100\% = 3.95\%$$

The result, 3.95%, falls within the acceptable range of quality costs established as the cost parameters. This calculation should be done for each department as part of its annual program evaluation. It should also be followed over time. In addition, quality costs for each department may be charted on a bar graph to provide a total cost picture. An average of the total quality costs percentages (TQCP) of all departments can be calculated to determine the mean quality costs percentage (MQCP) for the division of nursing.

$$\frac{\text{TQCP (department A) + TQCP (department B) + TQCP (department C), etc.}}{\text{Total number of departments}} = \text{MQCP (mean quality cost as a percentage of operating income for all departments within the division of nursing)}$$

It is important to keep in mind that these cost analyses are not budgeting allocations. These measures are used to identify how budgeted dollars have been spent on quality activities.

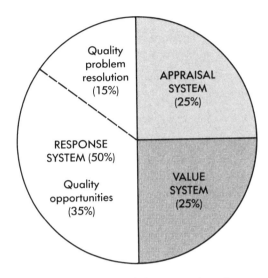

■ **FIGURE 15-2**   **Allocation of the costs of quality management.**

Quality costs can also be examined with respect to the costs associated with the value system, the appraisal system, and the response system.

Costs associated with the value system consist of the costs associated with developing the standards that serve as the basis for quality within the system and the cost of quality education. These two components include all quality awareness mechanisms within the organization. Examples of value-associated costs include the cost of staff time required to develop the standards and the cost of staff time required to develop and conduct educational programs related to quality in general and to specific standards.

Costs associated with the appraisal process are the costs of staff time and costs of materials expended to carry out the monitoring and evaluation activities. These may include the cost of developing and duplicating data collection forms, the cost of data collection, analysis and reporting, and any additional staffing required to complete the monitoring and evaluation activities.

Costs associated with the response system include costs of all those activities and materials that are necessary to correct a quality problem or take advantage of a quality opportunity. These might include the cost of council time to develop an action plan and the costs of labor and materials necessary to pilot the proposed change.

These three costs are associated with each important aspect of care/service being monitored by each department. Costs associated with the value system and those associated with the identification and development of quality opportunities represent the cost of prevention. Costs associated with the appraisal/assessment system are appraisal costs, and those associated with problem resolution include failure costs. When the focus is on quality improvement, the bulk of costs associated with quality should be spent on preventing problems and taking advantage of quality opportunities. The authors suggest that approximately 25% of the cost of quality be spent on developing the value system (standards development and education), 25% be spent on monitoring and evaluation, and 50% be spent on the response system. Of the 50% allocated to the response system, ideally no more than 15% should be spent on problem resolution, leaving at least 35% to be spent on seeking quality opportunities. Figure 15-2 illustrates the suggested allocation of quality management costs.

The costs associated with each of the three systems as a percentage of operating income can be calculated. The sum of these percentages then equals the percentage of your operating income spent on quality.

$$\frac{\text{Value system (\$)}}{\text{Operating income (\$)}} \times 100\% = 0.5\text{-}1.0\%$$

$$\frac{\text{Appraisal system (\$)}}{\text{Operating income (\$)}} \times 100\% = 0.5\text{-}1.0\%$$

$$\frac{\text{Response system (\$)}}{\text{Operating income (\$)}} \times 100\% = 1.5\text{-}2.5\%$$

Let us look at an example. For an annual nursing department operating income of $950,000, the calculated costs of standards development and quality education might be $8,000; the cost of appraisal may be $12,000 and the cost of quality improvement might add up to $18,000. The cost of the value system would be:

$$\frac{\$8,000}{\$950,000} \times 100\% = 0.84\%$$

The cost of the appraisal system would be:

$$\frac{\$12,000}{\$950,000} \times 100\% = 1.26\%$$

and the cost of quality improvement would be:

$$\frac{\$18,000}{\$950,000} \times 100\% = 1.89\%$$

In this example, the value and response systems are within the defined cost limits; however, the appraisal costs fall outside the acceptable limits. This means it is costing more to monitor quality in that clinical department than is desirable, and a process analysis should be conducted to evaluate and justify the variance. If the variance is not justified, an administrative plan to reduce appraisal costs should be developed. Perhaps too much monitoring is being done or the wrong level of personnel is appraising. Even though the total quality costs of the department (4.0%) are within the acceptable limits, this analysis enables you to identify whether the correct balance among quality awareness, appraisal, and response activities is maintained. By reducing appraisal costs, total quality costs could be reduced or additional dollars could be diverted to quality improvement activities. This is the essence of productivity management.

■ PRODUCTIVITY MANAGEMENT AND QUALITY MANAGEMENT: TWO SIDES OF THE SAME COIN?

Productivity is not a four-letter word. Yet, because it has been so closely associated with cost reduction, it suffers from a bad image. Visions of efficiency experts with stop watches, time-motion studies, and massive layoffs are conjured up by the mere mention of the word. Seidman and Skancke emphasize, however, that "unless you are measuring your productivity, you will not know whether you are on course, off course, or ready to crash."[17]

Simply defined, productivity is the relationship of the output of a system to its input. A more comprehensive definition of productivity is a measure of organizational performance, i.e., the interplay of efficiency and effectiveness. Efficiency compares inputs and outputs. Effectiveness measures the extent to which the desired outcomes are achieved. In a product-oriented business, both inputs and outputs are easily quantifiable. Ten pounds of flour and sugar may be needed to produce 500 cookies. A specified amount of wood and nails is required to produce a 3- × 5-foot bookshelf.

In the service sector, inputs and outputs are not so easily quantified. In health care, a service is used as soon as it is "produced." Unlike products, services cannot be inventoried. They cannot be produced and stockpiled for use when demand for services exceeds staff capabilities. Also, service organizations usually produce varied and complex outputs. The outputs (e.g., procedures, laboratory tests, and surgeries) are not homogeneous entities. For example, the process and outcomes of a procedure may vary considerably based on the patient's demographics, diagnosis, and prognosis.

Attempts have been made to incorporate these variables into the development of productivity measures specially designed for health care. Case-mix measurement methods have been developed to address these factors. The most familiar case-mix method is Diagnosis Related Groups (DRGs); however, other case-mix measurement strategies have arisen to supplant or modify the DRG method. These include patient severity indexing, disease staging, and patient management categories. Health care output then becomes "treated cases where treatment is a combination of services expected to result in a positive outcome given patient illness characteristics and the current state of knowledge."[7] Current trends in defining health care outputs increasingly emphasize the quality as well as the quantity of the output.

Inputs to the health care system include the labor and materials discussed earlier. Defining the outputs of a program and comparing them to the cost of the inputs enables you to analyze how much it costs to produce the results you achieved. When you assign a monetary value to the outputs, an estimate of "return on investment" can be made. For example, the actual cost savings achieved from implementing a quality improvement plan can be calculated and compared to the cost of producing that change. If the benefits outweigh the costs, the program is successful, but, if the costs exceed the benefits, the quality program should be carefully examined. Carroll argues, however, that determining costs related to quality programs in hospitals is difficult because of lack of uniformity in cost accounting methodologies related to quality expenses.[4] Also of significance is the fact that many hospitals include quality related activities as part of the expense of providing the regular duties of the nursing department. Thus, Carroll believes that recent published data on the cost of quality nationally are unreliable.[4] Correcting these discrepancies is necessary for accurate national trending. The first step is to develop a standardized quality cost accounting system that can be universally adopted.

While financial analysis provides a concrete perspective on the costs associated with quality, to view it as the sole determinant of success or failure is economic myopia. Sometimes the quality improvements are necessary regardless of the cost. Thus, additional indicators of the progress of the quality management program are needed.

■ MEASURING PRODUCTIVITY

The second indicator of the success of a quality program is its productivity. Edwardson describes four benefits of productivity measurement[7]:

1. It measures progress in goods/service.
2. It documents efficiency improvement.

3. It explains whether improvements are due to better design or process.
4. It provides a criterion for resource distribution.

Measuring productivity is useful to document progress in the production of goods and services. It answers questions about whether efficiency and effectiveness are improving. Are the resources (inputs) necessary to produce the results (outputs) appropriate and cost effective? Does increased monitoring and evaluation result in increased quality of care? Productivity measurement controls resource utilization. Finally, measuring current progress can generate further success.

Productivity measures abound. In baseball, statistics or "stats"—e.g., RBIs, ERAs, batting averages, and stolen bases—serve as productivity measures for a player or team. In the new ball game of health care, quality stats are a significant performance measurement. This is evidenced by the Joint Commission's Agenda for Change in which one of the major objectives is to develop a national performance data base against which individual institutions can measure their performance.[15]

No one instrument can measure productivity. Young encourages considering the following factors in developing a productivity measure[19]:

1. Scope and organization of the department
2. Staffing, scheduling, department layout, equipment
3. Working relationships between departments and the systems used within a department

These factors can negatively or positively affect productivity. The scope and organization of the division of nursing affect its performance. Chapters 4 and 5 discussed the shared governance system and scope of service. The successful utilization of the council structure will significantly affect quality productivity. Poor communication among councils, redundancy in efforts, or inappropriate utilization of council time will significantly reduce performance.

Staffing, scheduling, department layout, and equipment also influence quality productivity. Staff must be available to perform the tasks associated with quality such as attending council meetings, collecting data, and writing reports in addition to providing quality patient care. Staff members who worry about who is taking care of their patients while they attend a council meeting cannot be effective. The commitment of the extra resources (people, space, and equipment) necessary to carry out the work of quality management is essential. Without adequate tools, productivity suffers. Computers are the most important new tool to enhance productivity. "They provide information, control operations and monitor quality at a relatively low cost."[17]

Finally, interdepartmental relationships and operating systems affect productivity. Productivity measures are developed using productivity units. These units represent the average amount of input needed to produce a specific outcome. Examples of quality resources that might be translated into quality productivity units include hours of data collection, hours of data analysis, hours of developing indicators, and the like.

Seidman and Skancke also suggest that productivity measures should be simple. Intricate measurement systems can cost more to calculate than the worth of the data they provide.[17]

Traditional approaches to quantifying quality productivity include counting and summary methods. Counting methods are done for comparison. Examples include volume indicators such as how many studies were done this year as compared to last year. Summary methods analyze the impact of quality management on patient care. In this method, quality productivity is analyzed according to the numbers of resolved problems and/or the cost savings associated with producing the desired results. Effectiveness may be quantified by looking at the number of times the total number of outcomes in a specific department fell within the predetermined threshold parameters. For example, department A monitors outcome indicators for two critical aspects of care. Because these outcomes relate to critical aspects of care, they are monitored quarterly for a total of eight monitoring events. Suppose that of the eight monitoring events, all calculated thresholds fell within the predefined threshold parameters. The following equation might be used to determine the percentage of time in which a threshold for evaluation can be predicted with confidence:

$$100\% \times \frac{\text{No. of times calculated threshold falls within threshold parameters}}{\text{Total no. of monitoring events (annually)}}$$

or

$$100\% \times \frac{8}{8} = 100\%$$

This type of tracking is useful to substantiate a reduction in monitoring frequency. The total annual number of monitoring events is divided into the number of times the calculated threshold fell within the threshold parameters.

If only six of the eight monitoring events fell within the threshold parameters then the equation would be as follows:

$$100\% \times \frac{6}{8} = 75\%$$

In the first instance, the reviewer could say with confidence that 100% of the times monitored, the outcomes fell within the threshold parameters. However, in the second case, this happened only 75% of the time. By predetermining an acceptable standard for altering monitoring frequency, this equation can be used to set next year's monitoring schedule. For example, your monitoring standard may state that critical aspects of care are monitored at least quarterly (see Chapter 6); however, if over the course of a year (e.g., four monitoring events), 100% of the calculated thresholds fall within the threshold parameters, monitoring may be decreased to three times per year for the next calendar year. An additional standard must also be written to address readjustment of the frequency upward if the percentage drops below 100%.

Another measure of the effectiveness of the quality program might be the length of stay. Ideally, improved quality of care results in reduced length of stay. Zander describes the impact of the use of the critical path process on anticipated length of stay for Alliant Health System.[20] Tracking of indicators revealed:

Decreases	Increases
Length of stay (ALOS)	Total discharges
Charge/cost per case	Charge/cost per day
Patient days (relative to total discharges)	(greater acuity in fewer days)
Total charges/costs (relative to total discharges)	

Reduced length of stay expressed as cost savings is an important variable in analyzing whether the benefits of the quality program outweigh its costs. It is one type of monetary saving that results from improved quality.

Another direct benefit related to the quality program is the cost saving associated with streamlining the process of providing care while maintaining the quality of the outcomes. Zander, for example, projected reduction in charges of over $11 million for three hospitals, primarily resulting from length of stay reduction. Time, materials, and equipment saved can also be translated into calculable dollar income or savings. Quantifying these benefits makes it easier to compare them with costs and thus easier to make decisions about the allocation of resources.[20]

Productivity measures also include patient outcomes. A variety of scales are available to quantify patient problems.[2,11] These scoring systems attach a designated score to each patient problem, staging the problem from least severe to most severe. Internal scoring systems specific to an institution may also be developed based on the stages identified for a specific patient problem or nursing diagnosis. These rating scales can then be used to identify the numbers of patients in each category who achieved the desired outcomes for that problem. For example, an indicator might be as follows:

$$100\% \times \frac{\text{Total no. of patients with acquired stage IV pressure ulcer}}{\substack{\text{Total no. of patients with acquired stage IV pressure ulcers} \\ \text{who progressed to level III or above by discharge}}}$$

These equations are specific examples of a modification of Carroll's[4] productivity calculation:

$$100\% \times \frac{\text{No. of resolved problems}}{\text{Total no. of follow-up studies}}$$

This equation focuses only on problem resolution, however, and does not include the quality opportunities. A more representative approach to outcome productivity might be to add problem resolution and opportunity as follows:

$$100\% \times \frac{\substack{\text{No. of resolved problems} + \text{no. of quality opportunities} \\ \text{that yielded favorable results}}}{\text{Total no. of aspects studied}}$$

or

$$100\% \times \frac{\text{Total no. of successful quality improvements}}{\text{Total no. of important aspects monitored}}$$

The major disadvantage of cost-benefit analysis is that some benefits are not easily quantified in dollars and cents. These include such things as improved patient and staff satisfaction, which is why an additional type of indicator must be analyzed when evaluating quality management effectiveness.

■ PERCEIVED QUALITY: THE EYES OF THE BEHOLDER

In addition to identifying the financial benefits or outcomes of your quality management program, the intangible benefits must also be considered. No evaluation of the effects of quality improvement is complete without an analysis of the impact of the program on customer satisfaction. Customers of the quality program include patients, nursing staff, physicians, other departments, and administration. A thorough analysis of the satisfaction trends in these groups is necessary.

Satisfaction levels regarding the quality program itself should also be tracked. Satisfaction may be defined as the customer's perception of how the quality management program is operating. What effect does the quality programming have on their hospital stay, daily practice, department operations? What areas do they see as needing improvement and what strengths can they identify?

While much has been written on developing patient satisfaction tools and staff climate surveys, none specifically discuss the inclusion of questions related to the quality management program. As consumers, both patients and staff, become more knowledgeable about quality improvement, this type of survey will become an essential element of program review.

■ PROCESS REVIEW: HOW WELL IS THE QUALITY PROGRAM OPERATING?

The fourth and final area for analysis of the quality program is the process. Just as in clinical monitoring, procedures, practice guidelines, plans, and documentation are reviewed, quality processes must be evaluated for their efficiency.

The Joint Commission has outlined specific data elements related to the quality program. These include seven characteristics of departmental monitoring and evaluation activities:

These activities:
- Are planned, systematic, and ongoing
- Are comprehensive;
- Are based on indicators;
- Are accomplished by routine collection and periodic evaluation of data;
- Result in appropriate actions to resolve identified problems;
- Are continuous; and
- Are integrated.[14]

Planned, systematic, and ongoing means that there is a record of a written plan based on the ten-step process and that the evaluation activities occur over time rather than as a series of one-time studies. Comprehensive means that the monitoring and evaluation activities address both the quality and appropriateness of care provided by all levels of personnel. It also suggests that the studies include all major diagnostic,

---

NC.6 As part of the hospital's quality assurance program, the quality and appropriateness of the patient care provided by all members of the nursing staff are monitored and evaluated in accordance with Standard QA.3 and Required Characteristics QA.3.1 through QA.3.2.8 in the "Quality Assurance" chapter in this *Manual* (the *AMH*).

NC.6.1 The nurse executive is responsible for implementing the monitoring and evaluation process.

NC.6.1.1 Nursing staff members participate in

NC.6.1.1.1 the identification of the important aspects of care for each patient care unit;

NC.6.1.1.2 the identification of the indicators used to monitor the quality and appropriateness of the important aspects of care; and

NC.6.1.1.3 the evaluation of the quality and appropriateness of care.

NC.6.2 When an outside source(s) provides nursing services, the nurse executive, or the chief executive officer in the absence of a nurse executive, is responsible for implementing the monitoring and evaluation process.

■ FIGURE 15-3   Standard NC.6 of the Accreditation Manual for Hospitals.
(Copyright 1991 by the Joint Commission on Accreditation of Healthcare Organizations, Oakbrook Terrace, IL. Used with permission.)

therapeutic, and preventive functions of each department. Documentation of this would be found in each department's plan and individual studies. All monitoring and evaluation should be done using indicators developed from the important aspects of care/service that meet the characteristics of good indicators. Routine collection and periodic evaluation are carried out for each indicator that will adequately represent a true picture of quality for that indicator. Documentation of the intent to act to improve care, the actions taken, and the results of those actions is essential. Continuous monitoring means that evaluation continues for important aspects of care even after problem resolution. Finally, integration of the quality monitoring activities with other departmental and/or hospital-wide monitoring efforts is documented.

In addition to these generic characteristics, NC.6 of the *Accreditation Manual for Hospitals* outlines additional standards that must be adhered to (Figure 15-3). These include the role of the nurse executive in implementing the monitoring and evaluation process and nursing staff participation.[1]

Just as in clinical monitoring, quality program analysis should be concurrent. Evaluating key processes as they occur provides feedback for immediate quality improvement rather than waiting until year's end. Also, the focus must concentrate on the critical aspects of the quality program, i.e., step 3 of the ten-step process applied to the quality management service.

The Joint Commission has also established a task force on quality assessment to develop an incremental approach to continuous quality improvement. This task force has developed standards related to quality assessment and improvement which are included in the 1992 accreditation manuals and will further clarify the structure, process, and outcome of quality monitoring and improvement.

REFERENCES

1. Accreditation manual for hospitals, Chicago, 1992, Joint Commission on Accreditation of Health Care Organizations.
2. Allen RH: Use of the problem-oriented record to evaluate treatment in a chronic psychiatric population, Qual Assurance Bull 8(3): 13-16, 1982.
3. Burda D: Total quality management becomes big business, Modern Healthcare 21:25-29, 1991.
4. Carroll JG: Restructuring hospital quality assurance, Chicago, 1984, Dow Jones Irwin.
5. Crosby P: Quality is free, New York, 1979, McGraw-Hill Book Co.
6. Donabedian A: Five essential questions from the management of quality in health care, Health Manage Quart 9(1):6-9, 1987.
7. Edwardson S: Measuring nursing productivity, Nurs Econ 3(1):9-14, 1985.
8. Garvin D: Managing quality: the strategic and competitive edge, Glencoe, 1988, Free Press.
9. Israeli A and Fisher B: Cutting quality costs, Quality Progress 14(1):46-48, 1991.
10. Johnson J: Investors link quality of care to the bottom line, Hospitals 64(17):86, 1990.
11. Jones KR: Severity of illness measured systems: an update, Nurs Econ 5(6):292-296, 1987.
12. Juran J: Quality control handbook, ed 4, New York, 1988, McGraw-Hill Book Co.
13. Melum M: The next generation of health care quality, Hospitals 63:80, 1989.
14. Monitoring and evaluation in nursing services, Chicago, 1986, Joint Commission on Accreditation of Hospitals.
15. O'Leary D: President's column, Perspectives 9:1, 1989.
16. Puetz B: Evaluation in nursing staff development, Rockville, IL, 1985, Aspen Systems Corporation.
17. Seidman LW and Skancke SL: Productivity, New York, 1990, Simon and Schuster.
18. Walton M: The Deming management method, New York, 1986, Putnam Publishing Group.
19. Young LC and Hayne AN: Nursing administration: from concepts to practice, Philadelphia, 1988, WB Saunders.
20. Zander K: Estimating and tracking the financial impact of critical paths, Definition 5(4): 1-3, 1990.

16

IMPROVING YOUR
QUALITY MANAGEMENT PROGRAM

The road to success is always under construction.
ANTHONY ROBBINS

Alice thought she had never seen such a curious croquet-ground in her life: it was all ridges and furrows; the croquet balls were live hedgehogs, and the mallets live flamingoes, and the soldiers had to double themselves up and stand on their hands and feet, to make the arches.

The chief difficulty Alice found at first was managing her flamingo: she succeeded in getting its body tucked away, comfortably enough, under her arm, with its legs hanging down, but generally, just as she had got its neck nicely straightened out, and was going to give the hedgehog a blow with its head, it would twist itself round and look up into her face, with such a puzzled expression that she could not help bursting out laughing; and, when she had got its head down, and was going to begin again, it was very provoking to find that the hedgehog had unrolled itself, and was in the act of crawling away: besides all this, there was generally a ridge or a furrow in the way wherever she wanted to send the hedgehog to, and, as the doubled-up soldiers were always getting up and walking off to other parts of the ground, Alice soon came to the conclusion that it was a very difficult game indeed.

The players all played at once without waiting for turns, quarrelling all the while, and fighting for the hedgehogs; and in a very short time the Queen was in a furious passion and went stamping about, and shouting "Off with his head!" or "Off with her head!" about once a minute.

Alice began to feel very uneasy: to be sure, she had not as yet had any dispute with the Queen, but she knew that it might happen any minute, "and then," thought she, "what would become of me? They're dreadfully fond of beheading people here: the great wonder is, that there's any one left alive!"

She was looking about for some way of escape, and wondering whether she could get away without being seen, when she noticed a curious appearance in the air: it puzzled her very much at first, but after watching it a minute or two she made it out to be a grin, and she said to herself "It's the Cheshire-Cat: now I shall have somebody to talk to."

"How are you getting on?" said the Cat, as soon as there was mouth enough for it to speak with.

Alice waited till the eyes appeared, and then nodded. "It's no use speaking to it," she thought, "till its ears have come, or at least one of them." In another minute the whole head appeared, and then Alice put down her flamingo, and began an account of the game, feeling very glad she had someone to listen to her. The Cat seemed to think that there was enough of it now in sight, and no more of it appeared.

"I don't think they play at all fairly," Alice began, in rather a complaining tone, "and they all quarrel so dreadfully one can't hear oneself speak—and they don't seem to have any rules in particular; at least, if there are, nobody attends to them—and you've no idea how confusing it is all the things being alive: for instance, there's the arch I've got to go through next walking about at the other end of the ground—and I should have croqueted the Queen's hedgehog just now, only it ran away when it saw mine coming!"

"How do you like the Queen?" said the Cat in a low voice.

"Not at all," said Alice: "she's so extremely—" Just then she noticed that the Queen was close behind her, listening: so she went on "—likely to win, that it's hardly worth while finishing the game."*

Rapid changes in quality monitoring and evaluation in the field of health care are akin to Alice's croquet game. Just when you think you understand how to play the game and are in control of all the pieces and players, the game rules change and the pieces and players move. Just as Alice had trouble playing croquet amid rapid changes, so key players in the new game of quality must deal with constant change.

In the book *When Giants Learn to Dance,* Rosabeth Moss Kanter suggests that it is getting harder and harder to succeed with traditional corporate methods when technology, customer preferences, employee loyalty, industry regulations, and corporate ownership are constantly changing. "Instead of simply keeping their own eyes on the ball, they have to watch all the changing elements of the game at once." Winning requires "faster action, more creative maneuvering, more flexibility and closer partnership with employees and customers" than ever before.[8] Dennis O'Leary, MD, president of the Joint Commission says, "We have no small number of challenges facing us ahead." He was referring to the disorder in the evaluative and regulatory environment. "If problems are treasures, we are quite rich."[12]

Rosabeth Moss Kanter cites a 1986 survey of nearly 100 large corporations in which 83% had already devoted an average of 2.2 years to some sort of self-improvement campaign. At this point they are beyond the "exciting (and easy) inspirational/rhetorical/philosophical stage. They are facing tough questions about whether they really mean it." She believes some companies are stumbling over the roadblocks to improvement including resistance, cynicism, and the sheer fatigue of so much change. Executives are beginning to realize that "when everyone aspires to excellence it only makes the competition tougher; it does not guarantee business success."[8]

This chapter focuses on strategies to manage the dynamic nature of the quality management program. As we discussed in Chapter 14, the first phase of the quality management program sets the quality values for the organization. Phase two, described in Chapter 15, evaluates the efficiency and effectiveness of the quality management program. In other words, it is the appraisal of the quality management program itself. The response system is the third phase. It fosters continual improvement. It incorporates the values from phase one and data from phase two to determine what is working and what is not. It then attempts to fix whatever is not working and to refine what is. For example, evaluation of the data collection method used in phase two may reveal that the data collection form is cumbersome and confusing to staff and the accuracy of the data is being affected as a result. A corrective action plan would be developed that might include redesign of the form to simplify its use. Quality improvement is the phase that enables you to change the quality management program to find quicker, smarter, more cost-effective mechanisms for administering the quality program and ensuring quality results. Effective quality management within the quality department is critical to the implementation of a successful organization-wide quality management program.

---

*Excerpted from Carroll L: *Alice's Adventures in Wonderland and Through the Looking Glass,* Boston, 1980, GK Hall and Co.

■ THE SIX-STAGE PROCESS FOR QUALITY IMPROVEMENT

Excellence guru Tom Peters describes a six-stage process for quality improvement. These stages define an evolutionary process for the quality management department and delineate the progression from novice to expert. They suggest a quality management maturation process that defines quality improvement within the quality management department itself. These changes must take place if the organization is to thrive in tomorrow's health care environment.

Peters believes that while a few firms have attained bits and pieces of each of the six stages, none has yet established a scheme which includes all of them. "Getting to, and through, stages one and two is no mean feat; but it's not enough for survival."[14]

The six-stage quality improvement process that Peters outlines includes:

Stage 1: Conformance quality
Stage 2: Whose specs?
Stage 3: Perception is king
Stage 4: All to the customer
Stage 5: Teams with customers
Stage 6: No barriers, no borders

Stage 1 involves getting service process variance under control. It is internally oriented in its conformance quality, that is, it defines quality by the internal workings of the system and its workers. Stage 2 incorporates the customer's input into the design of specifications. In stage 3, attention is focused on the customer's perception of quality or the lack thereof. Stage 4 puts all functional areas of the company in touch with customers on a routine basis. Stage 5 makes customers full scale partners in conformance, quality improvement, process improvement, accounting-systems improvement, and product design. Finally, in stage 6, the barriers between the functions inside the firm and borders with outsiders are destroyed. As Tom Peters states, "I have an infuriating way of sketching organization charts these days. I simply draw a big circle on a flip chart and proclaim, 'Everybody in!'"[14]

While stage 6 is the ultimate goal of all quality programs, moving through the stages represents the process of continual improvement.

The whole quality field is evolving. The emphasis of quality improvement efforts in health care to date have been on patient care. There is a dearth of information regarding quality improvement in the quality program. Mechanisms to improve the efficiency and effectiveness of quality management activities free staff to spend more time in providing rather than monitoring patient care.

Dennis O'Leary writes, "While the direct care provided by physicians, nurses, and other clinicians is undeniably important, effective governance, management, and support services are equally important to the provision of good care."[10] The quality management program is an administrative support service. It provides administration with vital information about its performance relative to internal and externally defined quality indicators. As such, the performance of the quality management program has a significant impact on decisions that are made to chart the course of that institution. On-going, continuous improvement in the quality management program is critical.

Improvement, however, cannot be haphazard. It must be based on a statistical approach using the scientific tools described in Chapter 10 and the planning processes outlined in Chapter 11. Also, just as changes within the clinical, professional, and administrative domains must be based on research findings, improvements in quality management must also have a scientific basis. This knowledge base is growing by borrowing useful concepts and tools that were developed and tested in other industries and adapting them to the peculiarities of health care.

Potential problems that can affect the quality program are many: overmonitoring or undermonitoring, cumbersome data collection, inadequate sampling, untrained staff, lack of secretarial support, and poor communication are just a few examples. Quality opportunities, however, also abound. These may include opportunities for interdisciplinary monitoring, streamlining data collection, and enhancing the accuracy of evaluation processes.

There are three key strategies that are essential to improving the efficiency and effectiveness of the quality management program. They are developing a culture of quality, communicating about quality, and redefining the role of the quality professional in health care.

■ CREATING A CULTURE OF QUALITY

According to Deal and Kennedy, a culture is a "system of informal rules that spells out how people are to behave most of the time."[4] Employees should know exactly what is expected of them and should be able to comply without wasted time and effort.

Deal and Kennedy describe five key elements that make up a strong culture:

1. Business environment
2. Values
3. Heroes
4. Rites and rituals
5. Cultural network

These elements apply directly to the continual enculturalization of quality.

The business environment is the single greatest influence in shaping a corporate culture. The environment is which a company operates determines what it must do to be successful. Designing an environment for success will be discussed later in this chapter as the second strategy for successful quality improvement.

Values are the beliefs of the organization made explicit in their written standards. These standards must be well defined and disseminated throughout the organization. Chapter 14 discussed the development of quality standards for the quality management department.

Heroes are those people who personify the values of the organization and who are role models for employees to follow. The evolving role of the quality professional as a "hero" within the organization will be described later in this chapter. Managers and individual staff members can also be "heroes" and should be recognized as such.

Rites and rituals are the systematic routines of day-to-day life in the organization. They exemplify the behavior that is expected of employees and tangibly demonstrate what the company stands for. In terms of quality, these rites include the monitoring and evaluation activities that are a critical part of each individual's job. These rites and rituals may also be evidenced in the recognition systems that have been established to reward excellence.

Finally, the cultural network serves as the primary (but informal) means of communication within the organization. It is through the network that the true values are passed along from employee to employee and department to department. For example, Mary Jane Moon, RN, may have resigned with official notification of a new job offer. However, the truth according to the "grapevine" may be that Mary Jane made too many medication errors. Using this informal network can be a powerful method for communicating the vision of quality. For example it can be instrumental in changing the perception of monitoring and evaluation as "blame fixing."

"Culture causes organizational-inertia; it's the brake that resists change because this is precisely what culture should do—protect the organization from willy-nilly responses to fads and short term fluctuations."[4] Overcoming this inertia requires continuous effort over time. It cannot be accomplished merely by writing new standards. It has been the authors' experience that in moving to a culture of quality it takes approximately 2 years of consistent effort before overt signs of the new culture are evident. In the fast-paced world of health care where we are accustomed to seeing immediate results, this process can appear painfully slow. So slow, in fact, and so fraught with resistance and cynicism that like Alice and the croquet game, many people throw their hands up in desperation and quit the game. There is no substitute for time. Developing a culture of quality is analogous to running in a marathon. Those who persist, who pace themselves well, and have a long-range strategy will ultimately succeed.[4]

An effective strategy to develop a strong culture of quality requires three elements:

1. A top-down commitment
2. An environment to succeed
3. Quality education

A top-down commitment to quality is essential to the development and growth of a culture of quality. The new quality assessment and improvement standards developed by the Joint Commission for implementation in 1992 clearly define the role of leadership in setting the priorities for organization-wide quality improvement activities. The revisions are designed to emphasize the role of hospital leaders in quality improvement activities. In fact, the very first standard speaks to this.[1,6]

O'Leary states, "Leadership can make or break quality improvement efforts in an organization. These initiatives don't just happen; they do not bubble up from the grass roots; they move from the top down." He believes that continuous quality improvement (CQI) is an organization-wide way of life which is helpful to the organization and good for the patient whom it serves.[10]

Top-down commitment must be shown in everything that is done. In other words, management has to "walk like it talks." Without that consistency, staff will mistrust management and not take the quality initiative seriously. For example, if management extols the virtues of continuous quality improvement, but balks at spending the money for the needed changes, staff receives conflicting messages. Likewise, the nurse manager who constantly stresses the importance of responding to patient call bells but does not respond to staff "call bells" sends a mixed message about responding to customer requests.

Crosby suggests that a culture of quality requires faith in management and actions that support that faith. He suggests developing a corporate policy on quality to make it clear that the commitment is real. He also recommends that quality be made the standing first item on management meeting agendas and that management continually reaffirm to staff the vision of quality and the way in which that commitment is being realized.[3]

The vision of quality, however, is like a seed. If it falls on barren ground, it will lie there and remain a seed. If it is watered and fertilized, it germinates and becomes a strong seedling. That seedling needs constant nourishment and the proper environment if it is to survive and flourish. So too, the quality management program itself needs a supportive environment for its potential to be fully realized. Quality improvement efforts in the quality management program focus on the development and maintenance of a professional practice environment. This involves participatory decision-making through controlled decentralization that promotes a sense of accountability in individuals for achieving the organization's goals and objectives.

The new quality improvement environment in organizations must be one of security and not fear and one that promotes communication rather than isolation. Deming insists that it is essential to drive out fear: "People are afraid to point out problems for fear they will start an argument, or worse, be blamed for the problem."[17] An environment that utilizes quality monitoring to affix blame cannot support a quality management program. That type of environment only fosters deception and mistrust. Porter-O'Grady states that "workers begin to build trust immediately upon joining an organization, expecting a sharing of information that affects their personal and economic welfare. When the hospital does not honestly and freely supply all of the information workers need to do their jobs and to make judgments about their future there, a feeling of basic mistrust insidiously begins to undermine all other supports."[15] An environment of trust encourages the open exchange of information throughout the division of nursing. This environment enables participatory decision-making and provides staff with the information needed to make informed decisions. While staff members are held accountable for their decisions, the environment is free of reprisal and unwarranted disciplinary action. Risks are managed and there is freedom to fail. Dennis O'Leary believes ". . . there is a lot more to be gained by improving the norm than by punishing all of the outliers."[9]

No one can feel comfortable in an environment that does not provide the material and fiscal support necessary for staff to act responsibly upon decisions. A fertile environment for quality involves valuing staff's administrative responsibilities for monitoring and improving the results of nursing care as much as it values the provision of that care. Staff should be free from clinical responsibilities when attending to their quality responsibilities without the need for worry about who is caring for their patients while they are out of the department. Administration must ensure staff are able to carry out monitoring and evaluation activities as part of their routine job responsibilities, not as an additional task for them to "fit in" as time permits. Commitment of resources to support the quality functions of the division enhances staff trust in the quality rhetoric and translates it to reality. Commitment of resources also involves recognizing quality efforts and rewarding quality accomplishments. A strong recognition program is necessary to keep the fires of staff enthusiasm for the quality program burning brightly and motivates staff to even higher levels of excellence.

To participate in this new quality environment in a meaningful way, staff members must be fluent in the language and processes of quality. Learning a foreign culture begins with a familiarization with the language and rituals or customs of the country; so too, in the unfamiliar world of quality improvement, staff must have an opportunity to acclimate. A solid educational curriculum for quality is essential at all levels throughout the nursing division. The Joint Commission's 1992 quality assessment and improvement standards emphasize the necessity of training staff to assess and improve processes that contribute to better patient outcomes.[1,6] Education regarding quality includes training in terminology, data collection, statistical analysis, decision making, strategic planning, and change. The depth and scope of the quality training are based on position responsibilities. For example, nursing assistants may be involved in data collection, while registered nurses would be responsible for data analysis and interpretation. Both groups however would need to know the basic, or core, terminology. The educational process is ongoing; it begins with orientation and continues throughout the staff member's tenure within the division of nursing. To be meaningful, the information must be repeated periodically to reinforce the message and update staff as to the latest changes taking place at the national, regional, local, and institutional levels.

The provision of an environment for success and the development of quality education are closely linked to the introduction of technology that will enable staff to collect, process, analyze, and project trends in large volumes of information quickly and efficiently. Computer technology can greatly facilitate quality activities and education. Its successful implementation requires that staff becomes literate in yet another language and culture, that of automated information processing. Unless staff members have the knowledge and skills necessary to use computer technology, its use can waste their time and energy. Used appropriately, however, computer technology is the key to taming the paper tiger of quality monitoring and evaluation.

■ INFORMATION SYSTEMS

In the late 1960s and 1970s, the world embraced computer technology and hailed it as a way to contain the rising costs of business and manufacturing. The health care industry also saw the possibilities of the new technology. Hospitals were quick to view computerization and automation as a solution to labor-intensive, hand-recorded, billing systems. Early computers primarily facilitated basic arithmetic activities. For this reason, hospitals were eager to install computer systems and do away with the human error inherent in manual billing processes. Notwithstanding the enormous cost of early computer systems, trustees, administrators, and physicians saw the long-term benefits and cost savings of the initial large capital expenditure. Most saw the purchase and utilization of computers "as indications of their hospital's sophistication and progress."[5] Dennis O'Leary believes that manual data collection resulted in numerous errors, omissions, and incorrectly entered data elements.[11]

At present there is an enormous market for information systems software in the health care industry. Indeed, in today's quality environment, it is almost impossible to carry out quality management strategies and improve quality in a health care organization without automation. Just as tabulation by hand in payroll and billing systems has become obsolete, so manual data tabulation in the quality management department has become outdated. Today, quality improvement is most easily achieved in an environment of automation. Furthermore, as a national data base for quality information to be managed by the Joint Commission looms on the horizon, forward-looking organizations have started to prepare themselves for twenty-first century automation of quality data.

In fact, standard NC.5.5.1 of the Joint Commission's nursing care standards states, "The use of efficient interactive information management systems for nursing, other clinical (for example, dietary, pharmacy, physical therapy), and non-clinical information is facilitated wherever appropriate."[1] Also, at present, pilot hospitals involved in testing the Joint Commission's obstetrical indicators are learning to use new software developed by the Joint Commission to collect the data. "Since early 1989, pilot hospitals have been transmitting data to the Commission via floppy discs. Use of the obstetrics software has cut the cost and time of data collection by nearly 50 percent, as compared with the earlier manual approach."[2]

Some organizations, however, hesitate to extend computerization to their quality management departments. As one CEO explained to the authors, "We've been getting along just fine for years with a QA coordinator using a paper and pencil and I don't see any reason for such a big expense now." Despite the obvious advantages, there are many concerns with automating the quality management department. Some of these concerns include: cost, patient and staff confidentiality, and legal issues.

Cost

The initial investment in a hospital information system is undeniably great. The CEO who expressed concern for "such a big expense" was correct—the expense is great. However, he was short-sighted in not foreseeing the potential benefit and long-term cost savings to his organization. Many forward-looking organizations are making the investment. According to Schulz and Johnson, "Computer applications have increased substantially during the 1980's. Moreover, medical information systems are being developed rapidly. For example, a total hospital information system (HIS) was developed at El Camino Hospital in Mountain View, California. Evaluation of this system documented improved quality of care and increased productivity of the nursing staff. With continued advances in information gathering, storage, analysis, and retrieval, it is likely that HIS and similar programs will have a major impact on hospital operations in the decade ahead."[16]

In today's environment, quality improvement cannot occur without information systems that incorporate statistical approaches to data collection and analysis and that allow quality changes to be rapidly tracked. In many respects, a health care organization today cannot afford *not* to automate their quality management program. Organizations unwilling to provide resources to update their quality departments will find that they have not kept pace with the forward thrust of the Joint Commission's Agenda for Change.

Patient and Staff Confidentiality

Many health care organizations are concerned that patient and staff privacy, confidentiality of patient and staff information, and security of patient and staff data are threatened by computer technology. Privacy issues concern who controls patient and staff information, who ensures freedom from intrusion into patients' and staff's private data, and who prohibits misuse of information. A health professional's duty has traditionally included an obligation to safeguard the confidentiality of information collected, stored, transmitted, and retrieved in the health care system.[5]

With a computerized system, confidentiality may, in fact, be more carefully safeguarded than in traditional manual systems. With computerization, sensitive patient and staff data can be coded to allow access only to approved personnel who are given the code. Thus, the information can be made secure and patient and staff privacy is maintained.

Legal Issues

Hospitals are understandably wary of disseminating potentially incriminating data that have traditionally been safeguarded on incident reports. Incorporating these data into a national data bank of information might make them vulnerable to "discovery" by a plaintiff attorney taking legal action against the hospital.

Eskildson and Yates comment on the difference between industrial and health care data. "Aware of the importance of rapid feedback, leading industrial firms widely disseminate a broad range of data, particularly current quality findings and recent trends . . . many of the data are publicly posted for everyone to see. . . . Frequently both the firm's own quality data and those of its competitors are distributed and compared. The purpose is to generate and maintain a high level of wide-spread interest in prevention and improvement."[7]

Health care quality assessment findings, however, are typically closely guarded and given extremely limited distribution. The rationale for restricting access to the information is to limit vulnerability to legal discovery. The largely unrecognized drawback, however, is that in practice this policy also makes it more difficult to recognize and eliminate problems, thereby increasing the risk of adverse outcomes (and the subsequent legal repercussions) in the long run. Resolving this quandary will require creative rethinking of how to automate and protect data and internal discussions from legal discovery.[7]

Concerns about costs, patient confidentiality, and legal issues must be taken seriously; nevertheless, the path to progress lies in implementing computerized information systems. Quality professionals will have a much greater role to play in the future of health care if they take advantage of information systems. Quality management is far more complex than quality assurance because it involves every aspect of an organization and is constantly evolving and changing. If quality improvement is to be an ongoing process, then quality professionals must be trained to use information systems to their capacity.

A significant part of the success experienced in industry has come from using the tools of statistical process control (discussed in Chapter 10) to gather and interpret data to support fact-based decision making.[13] Quality professionals also must be taught to use these tools and apply them to variance data to support fact-based decisions in health care. However, automated systems must be in place to aid the professional in using statistical process control tools if health care is to keep pace with the great strides being made in quality in industry.

Automating the process of quality management within health care organizations may help remove the traditional punitive climate of QA. When a QA coordinator no longer "polices" staff, the negative quality environment may disappear as all staff members become intricately involved in the process of quality, entering their individual data at their computer terminals on a daily basis. This will provide a more balanced approach with structured, automated participation in information gathering and analysis from frontline staff who possess invaluable knowledge about problems and potential solutions.

Computerization will also be the key to interhospital and intrahospital comparison of data. At present, no baseline data exist between organizations as benchmarks for comparison. Indeed, such benchmarks will never exist unless automated, anonymous reporting systems are devised. Just as "polite" families never divulge family secrets hospitals will never divulge "hospital secrets," unless there is a risk-free environment in which to do so.

Personal computers and microcomputers are gaining popularity with quality professionals. They have the potential to totally transform quality aspects of health care organizations. For example, the computer-generated quarterly report may acquire a whole new look. Instead of several pages of narrative information, it may be a graphic report using bar or pie charts to display data visually.

Computer graphics capabilities will facilitate using a scientific approach routinely to create flow charts, work flow diagrams, and cause and effect diagrams and to use them for directed discussions to aid in problem solving.

Word processing applications on main frames, networking, and disk sharing will introduce a different kind of communication as will telefax capabilities and modems. For example, an electrocardiogram taken from a patient in the coronary care department complaining of chest pain may immediately be telefaxed directly to a physician in the office or at home who can read it, make a diagnosis, and issue orders. Modems also facilitate instant communication. A nurse caring for a patient for whom an unfamiliar drug has been prescribed may wonder about possible interactions with the other medications that are already prescribed for the patient. Using a modem, the nurse could call a computerized pharmacy library to check the drug's compatibility parameters and receive the information instantly on the computer screen.

In addition, spreadsheet and statistics software will enable all quality professionals to develop and use skills previously considered unattainable. In short, applications software packages adapted to quality functions are becoming more sophisticated and broader in scope and are available for word processing, data base management, graphics, project management, desktop publishing, communications/productivity tools, statistics, and the like in many configurations and a range of prices.

The outcome of the automation of quality management is increased speed of data collection, analysis, and reporting. It also generates more accurate data for decision making and enhances the potential for better organization-wide record keeping.

■ REDEFINING THE ROLE OF THE QUALITY PROFESSIONAL

The advent of information technology will have a profound impact on the quality professional. The traditional role of the quality assurance professional as a "numbers cruncher" is being replaced by a much broader role.

An accountant is responsible for the organization's financial health. He or she is not merely a "bean counter." Likewise, the quality professional of the future will not be a "problem counter," but rather will assume responsibility for the health of the division's quality program. The nursing quality assurance professional will become the nursing quality manager. In that leadership role, the nursing quality manager provides input at the highest level of nursing administration regarding the impact of decisions on the quality of services provided and should be an appointed member of the nursing executive council. Also the nursing quality manager serves as a role model to the staff. He or she becomes a "hero" who helps create a culture of quality as discussed earlier. According to Deal and Kennedy, as a quality hero, the nursing quality manager personifies the organization's values and epitomizes the strength of the organization. Heroes are ordinary people who accomplish extraordinary results. They show how the ideal of success lies within human capacity. They set the standard for performance and provide a lasting influence within the organization. "Heroes are concerned with the set of beliefs and values they hold and in making sure these beliefs and values are inculcated in the people around them."[4]

The challenge that faces quality management professionals as heroes is to shift the focus of their efforts from problem identification to improving the norm of performance, not only in patient care but within the staff, the system, and even the quality management department itself. Thus, the focus of the role of the quality management professional is changing dramatically from one of "problem counter" to one of coordinator and facilitator of change.

The quality manager must be able to lead the change to quality-based performance. He or she must move the organization forward by coordinating the efforts of all the departments within the division and facilitating the personal and collaborative growth necessary to foster continuous quality improvement.

Porter-O'Grady lists 11 points characterizing a change agent. A change agent needs to[15]:

1. Be the link between the organization's goals and objectives and the participants who will carry them.
2. Be a resource to those involved in the decision-making process.
3. Define and outline the planning processes essential to complete the work of the organization.

4. Be a stimulus to information gathering and to assessment of the varying components of change.
5. Be a continuing catalyst and energizer for maintaining the change momentum.
6. Assess the varying changes in the demand and flow of components of the process.
7. Be sensitive to the impact of change events on individuals and on the work group as a whole.
8. Be a communication link between the work group and the other individuals involved in the change process.
9. Be a conflict identifier, mediator, and resolution facilitator.
10. Be a stimulator of discussion, identifying new and creative ways to move the process forward.
11. Be a facilitator of problem-solving strategies when difficulties arise in advancing the changes.*

Perhaps a better title for the position may be "quality coach" for just as a coach instills confidence, enthusiasm, and commitment in a team, so the quality management professional rallies the health care team to work together to score the "big one."

■ CRITICAL COMPETENCIES FOR THE QUALITY MANAGER

This exciting new role for the quality professional is at the forefront of the organization's struggle to compete in today's tough health care race. For most organizations, a full-time quality manager is required to achieve the organization's goals. This new quality manager must devote all of his or her attention to the quest for continual improvement. To be effective in the position, the quality manager must possess 12 critical competencies:

1. Proficiency in the scientific approach
2. Currency in accreditation requirements and processes
3. Computer literacy
4. Critical thinking and problem solving abilities
5. Strong negotiation skills
6. Sales and marketing skills
7. Assertiveness
8. Ability to organize information, people, and resources
9. Ability to work collaboratively with and through others
10. Strong writing skills
11. Strong presentation skills
12. Team building skills

The evolving role of the quality manager is one of facilitator, coordinator, and integrator of those processes that provide the organization with quantitative information about the existence of quality within its service and ways to improve the effectiveness and efficiency of that service. Never before in the history of health care has a position served a more critical function.

---

*Reprinted from *Creative Nursing Administration* by T. Porter-O'Grady, p. 106, with permission of Aspen Publishers, Inc. © 1986.

Ultimately, quality improvement in the quality management department is essential to achieving quality within the nursing service. Quality improvement efforts must consistently strive to make the quality management program a standards-based system that emphasizes outcome achievement and process efficiency. This system incorporates quality as part of everyone's job and simplifies the process of monitoring quality within that job. Furthermore, this system focuses on priorities of performance and strives for continual improvement of service related to those priorities.

The pursuit of excellence is, in the words of a popular song, a long and winding road. This book has attempted to provide a bridge that connects the old road of quality assurance to the new one of quality management. It provides the signposts to direct you on a successful journey and should be a worthwhile companion along the way. However, the book alone is merely words on paper. It shares with you the authors' road map for success. The rest is up to you. In the words of Shel Silverstein,

> This bridge will only take you halfway there
> To those mysterious lands you long to see:
> Through gypsy camps and swirling Arab fairs
> And moonlit woods where unicorns run free.
> So come and walk awhile with me and share
> The twisting trails and wondrous worlds I've known.
> But this bridge will only take you halfway there—
> The last few steps you'll have to take alone.*

REFERENCES

1. Accreditation Manual for Hospitals, Chicago, 1992, Joint Commission for Health Care Organizations.
2. Agenda for Change Update, vol 3, no 2, Chicago, 1989, Joint Commission on Accreditation of Health Care Organizations.
3. Crosby PB: Quality without tears, New York, 1984, McGraw-Hill Book Co.
4. Deal TE and Kennedy AA: Corporate cultures, Reading, Mass, 1982, Addison-Wesley Publishing Co.
5. Delaney C: Computer technology. In McCloskey J and Grace HK, eds: Current issues in nursing, St Louis, 1990, CV Mosby Co.
6. Draft of 1992 Quality Assessment and Improvement Standards, Chicago, 1991, Joint Commission on Accreditation of Health Care Organizations.
7. Eskildson L and Yates GR: Lessons from industry: revising organizational structure to improve health care quality assurance, Quality Rev Bull 17(2):38-41, 1991.
8. Kanter RM: When giants learn to dance, New York, 1989, Simon and Schuster.
9. O'Leary D: Accreditation in the quality improvement mold—a vision for tomorrow, Quality Rev Bull 17(3):72-77, 1991.
10. O'Leary D: CQI—a step beyond QA, Quality Rev Bull 17(1):4-5, 1991.
11. O'Leary D as quoted by Koska M: JCAHO: Pilot hospitals' input updates Agenda for Change, Hospitals, pp 50-54, January 5, 1990.
12. O'Leary D as quoted by Ruark-Hearst M: Cornerstones of health care in the nineties: key constituencies debate propositions for collaborating in the quality revolution, Quality Rev Bull 17(2):60-65, 1991.
13. Orkin FI: Computers and quality. In Juran JM, editor: Juran's quality control handbook, ed 4, New York, 1988, McGraw-Hill Co.
14. Peters T: The quality progression: getting beyond the obvious, Enterprise on Line 1:2, 1991.
15. Porter-O'Grady T: Creative Nursing Administration, Rockville, 1986, Aspen Publishers.
16. Schulz R and Johnson AC: Management of hospitals and health services, ed 3, St Louis, 1990, CV Mosby Co.
17. Walton M: Deming management at work, New York, 1990, GP Putnam's Sons.

GLOSSARY

Accreditation The act of granting approval to an organization by an official review board after the organization has met specific written requirements or standards.

Administrative action plan A process standard that outlines a critical area for action, desired outcomes, required activities, and a timeline directed at improving organizational performance.

Agenda for Change The Joint Commission's multiyear initiative designed to reshape the accreditation process by improving the methods used by the Joint Commission to evaluate and monitor health care organizations.

AHCPR (The Agency for Health Care Policy and Research) Created in December 1989, the eighth agency of the federal government's public health service designed to enhance the quality of patient care through improved knowledge that can be used in meeting society's health care needs; AHCPR activities include developing clinically relevant practice guidelines.

Alpha testing The initial phase of field testing of indicators.

Appropriateness The degree to which the correct service is provided given the current state of knowledge.

THE BLUEPRINT A comprehensive quality management model that focuses on quality awareness, quality appraisal, and quality improvement in three domains of practice, clinical, professional, and administrative.

Case-mix "Relative frequency of different diagnoses or conditions among patients" (Joint Commission).*

Cause and effect diagram A statistical process control tool that depicts every factor that may influence a given process; it is popularly called a "fishbone" diagram because of its shape.

Clinical action plan A process standard that outlines a critical area for action, desired outcomes, required activities, and a timeline directed at improving patient care.

Common cause variance A minor variation in performance that is the result of chance occurrence(s) involving the patient, staff, or system that cannot be controlled.

Compliance A positive factor that signifies adherence or conformance to written standards; it is composed of those controllable patient, staff, and system factors that affect quality.

Continuous quality improvement The process of ongoing, systematic refinement of service delivery that is achieved through identification and correction of quality problems and/or the identification and exploitation of quality opportunities.

Control chart A statistical process control tool consisting of a run chart with statistically determined upper and lower limits drawn on either side of the process average.

Controlled decentralization Distribution among specific individuals and/or groups of the authority, responsibility, and accountability for clinical, professional, and administrative decisions, based primarily on the individual's or group's areas of expertise.

Control limits (See Threshold parameters.)

---

*Definitions designated Joint Commission are reprinted from the *Primer on Indicator Development and Application.* Copyright 1990 by the Joint Commission on Accreditation of Healthcare Organizations, Oakbrook Terrace, IL. Used with permission.

Cost-benefit analysis The evaluation of the relationship between the resources necessary to complete a project and the results obtained from its completion.

Council A group of individuals charged with a specific ongoing function within an organization.

Critical aspect of care An aspect of care that is high volume, high risk, problem prone, and high cost.

Data element "A single piece of information required by an indicator, subsequently aggregated in a manner with other data elements to identify indicator event occurrences" (Joint Commission).*

Demographic data Patient, staff, or system variables that may influence the results of monitoring a specific indicator.

Domain One of the three distinct areas of nursing practice—clinical practice, professional practice, and administrative practice.

Effectiveness The degree to which desired results are produced.

Efficiency The act of producing output with the minimum of waste, expense, or unnecessary effort; the ratio of useful output to the total input in any system.

Employee development plan A process standard that outlines a critical area for development, desired outcomes, required activities, and a timeline for completion directed at improving an individual staff member's performance.

Evaluation (1) The mechanisms by which a service will be monitored and including quality assessment, customer satisfaction, and research.

(2) "The review and assessment of the quality and/or appropriateness of an important aspect of care for which a pre-established level of performance (threshold for evaluation) has been reached during monitoring activities. The review and assessment may include peer review, pattern analysis, and/or trend analysis and is de-

signed to determine whether there is a problem and/or opportunity to improve care, and if so, to develop a plan of action to address the identified problem or opportunity to improve care."†

Extremely important aspect of care An aspect of care that is any combination of three of the four important aspects, i.e., high-volume, high-risk, problem-prone, and/or high-cost.

Fishbone diagram (See Cause and effect diagram.)

Flow chart A statistical process control tool that schematically diagrams the steps in a process.

Histogram A statistical process control tool used to depict frequency of occurrence. (See Pareto chart.)

Important aspects of care High-volume, high-risk, high-cost, or problem-prone clinical activities that directly affect the quality of patient care delivered.

Important aspects of governance High-volume, high-risk, high-cost, or problem-prone aspects of the system that directly affect the quality of patient care delivered.

Important aspects of practice High-volume, high-risk, high-cost, or problem-prone professional activities that directly affect the quality of patient care delivered.

Indicator "A measurement tool used to monitor and evaluate the quality of important governance, management, clinical, and support functions" (Joint Commission).*

Indicator information set "An aggregate of information about an indicator including the indicator statement, definition of terms, identification of the indicator type, rationale for use of the indicator, description of the indicator population, indicator data collection logic, and delineation of underlying factors that may explain variations in indicator data" (Joint Commission).*

---

*Definitions designated Joint Commission are reprinted from the *Primer on Indicator Development and Application.* Copyright 1990 by the Joint Commission on Accreditation of Healthcare Organizations, Oakbrook Terrace, IL. Used with permission.

†This definition is reprinted from the Joint Commission Glossary of Quality Assurance Terms which appears in Carole H. Patterson's "Standards of Patient Care: The Joint Commission Focus on Nursing Quality Assurance" in *Nursing Clinics of North America,* vol 23, no 3. Copyright 1988 WB Saunders Company, Philadelphia, PA. Used with permission.

Joint Commission on Accreditation of Health Care Organizations (Joint Commission) A private, voluntary, nonprofit, nongovernmental agency that was founded in 1951 as The Joint Commission on Accreditation of Hospitals (JCAH). It surveys and accredits hospitals and other health care organizations according to its published consensus standards.

Monitoring The planned, systematic, ongoing collection, compilation, and organization of data about an indicator of the quality and/or appropriateness of an important aspect of care, practice or governance, and the comparison of those data to a preestablished range of performance (threshold parameters) to determine the need for further investigation.

Outcome The results of service delivery including patient, staff, and organizational performance.

Pareto chart A statistical process control tool used to determine and visually depict frequencies and priorities.

Policy A structure standard that defines the clinical, professional, and administrative rules of an organization.

Practice guideline A written process standard for client care management that has the potential for improving the quality of clinical and consumer decision making; it "includes assessment and diagnosis, planning, intervention, evaluation and outcome" (ANA)‡; "a descriptive tool or standardized specification(s) for care of the 'typical' patient in the 'typical' situation" (Joint Commission)*; "a systematically developed statement to assist practitioner and patient decisions about appropriate health care for specific clinical circumstances" (AHCPR); also sometimes called a protocol or practice parameter.

Procedure A series of recommended actions for the completion of a specific clinical, professional, or administrative task.

Process The manner in which service will be delivered. Procedures, practice guidelines/protocols, action plans, and documentation systems describe process.

Productivity The process of yielding favorable, desirable, or useful results.

Protocol (See Practice guideline.)

Quality "The degree to which patient care services increase the probability of desired patient outcomes and reduce the probability of undesired outcomes given the current state of knowledge" (Joint Commission).*

Quality appraisal The second component of quality management, which consists of specific evaluation activities that determine conformance to the value system; also referred to as quality assessment or quality assurance.

Quality assessment (See Quality appraisal.)

Quality assurance (See Quality appraisal.)

Quality awareness The first component of quality management, which consists of the value system of the organization expressed as written standards.

Quality improvement The third component of quality management, which consists of the response mechanisms initiated to correct problems or take advantage of opportunities to improve the efficiency or effectiveness of clinical, professional, or administrative services.

Quality management A comprehensive management approach that focuses on the systematic, ongoing, and continuous awareness, monitoring, and improvement of quality in clinical, professional, and administrative practice.

Rate-based event A clinical, professional, or administrative occurrence for which a certain rate of occurrence is expected when state of the art care is provided. Investigation is required when the rate at which the event occurs exceeds a preset threshold.

Reliability The ability of a data-gathering device to obtain consistent results.

Run chart A statistical process control tool used to document the frequency with which an event occurs over a period of time.

Scope of care/service The range of care or service provided by an organization, depart-

---

*Definitions designated Joint Commission are reprinted from the *Primer on Indicator Development and Application.* Copyright 1990 by the Joint Commission on Accreditation of Healthcare Organizations, Oakbrook Terrace, IL. Used with permission.

‡This definition is reprinted from *The American Nurse,* vol 23, no 3. Copyright 1991 by the American Nurses Association. Used with permission.

ment, or service, including conditions treated, managed, or prevented, treatments provided, procedures used, populations served, locations where care or service are provided, times when care or services are provided, and professional disciplines and specialties providing services. The delineation of the scope of care or service is the basis for identifying the important aspects of care, practice, and governance on which monitoring and evaluation are focused.

Sentinel event A serious clinical, professional, or administrative occurrence that always requires investigation.

Shared governance An organized, systematic approach to decision making that enables all levels of nurses to participate in the resolution of clinical, professional, and administrative practice issues.

Special cause variance A variation in performance that occurs as a result of patient, staff, or system variables that can be controlled.

Staff development plan A process standard that outlines a critical area for development, desired outcomes, required activities, and a timeline for completion directed at improving the performance of more than one staff member.

Standard A written value defining the rules, actions, results, or analyses that are related to the patient, staff, or system and are sanctioned by an authority.

Standard deviation A measure of the dispersion of a frequency distribution that is the square root of the variance.

Standard of care A written value statement that defines the rules, actions, or conditions that direct patient care.

Standard of governance A written value statement that defines the rules, actions, and conditions that direct institutional or departmental functions.

Standard of practice A written value statement that defines the rules, actions, or conditions that direct the maintenance of professional status and credibility.

Statistical control A state in which the results of monitoring an important aspect of care

fall consistently within the threshold parameters but without an obvious trend or pattern.

Statistical process control The application of statistical techniques to the control of processes.

Structure The circumstances under which a service will be delivered; the organization's mission, philosophy, goals and policies define its structure.

Tampering Attempts to fix minor variations in performance that are due to chance; it usually results in wildly fluctuating variations that overcorrect or undercorrect a variation.

Ten-step process The steps defined by the Joint Commission that outline the specific activities involved in the monitoring and evaluation process.

Threshold (for evaluation) "The level at which a stimulus is strong enough to signal the need for organization response to indicator data and the beginning of the process of determining why the threshold has been crossed" (Joint Commission).

Threshold parameters The upper and lower limits of threshold acceptance that establish an acceptable range of compliance or noncompliance.

Trending Analyzing the results of numerous studies on the same indicator to identify patterns that may influence the quality of outcomes related to the important aspect of care or service being monitored.

Trifocus approach A strategy for monitoring and evaluation that considers all three domains of practice: clinical, professional, and administrative.

Validity An instrument's ability to actually measure or test what it is intended to measure or test.

Variation A difference in performance related to an important aspect of care; it may result from controllable or uncontrollable factors.

Very important aspect of care An aspect of care that is any combination of two of the four important aspects of care, i.e., high-volume, high-risk, problem-prone, and high-cost.

INDEX

NOTE: Page numbers in italics indicate boxed or illustrated material.

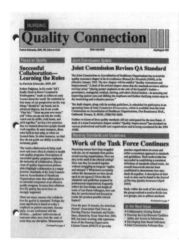
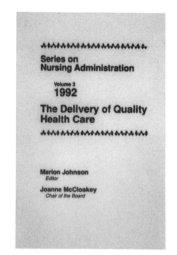
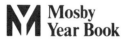